# nice
# dreads

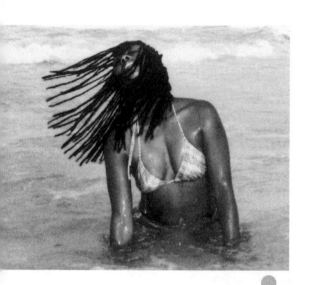

# nice
# dreads

Hair Care Basics and Inspiration for Colored
Girls Who've Considered Locking Their Hair

## Ionnice brittenum bonner

 THREE RIVERS PRESS • NEW YORK

Published in the United States by Three Rivers Press,
an imprint of the Crown Publishing Group,
a division of Random House, Inc., New York.
www.crownpublishing.com

THREE RIVERS PRESS and the Tugboat design are registered trademarks of
Random House, Inc.

Library of Congress Cataloging-in-Publication Data

Bonner, Lonnice Brittenum.
  Nice dreads : hair care basics and inspiration for colored girls who've
considered locking their hair / Lonnice Brittenum Bonner.—1st ed.
      p.  cm.
  1. African American women—Health and hygiene.  2. Hairdressing of
African Americans.  3. Hairdressing of Blacks.  4. Hair—Care and
hygiene.  5. Beauty, Personal.  6. Dreadlocks.  I. Title.

  RA778.4.A36B663   2005
  646.7'24'08996073—dc22

2004016265

ISBN 1-4000-5169-X

Printed in the United States of America

Design by Debbie Glasserman

10 9 8 7 6 5 4 3

First Edition

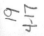

For Roland

# acknowledgments

My heartfelt thanks to all the people who supported me
with their creative contributions or who encouraged me
with pointed e-mails and remarks about the state of nappiness and my absence from the dialogue.

Barbara Lowenstein, Becky Cabaza, Orly Trieber, and
   Norman Kurz
The Right Prophetess Lisa Jones and Mr. Kenneth Brown
Gordon Eriksen and Heather Johnston—a special and
   heartfelt thanks for your incredible support of my vision
Aurelio José Barrera, Laura Mucel, and Steve Roberts

Capril Bonner-Thomas, Maya Bonner-Thomas, and Vea
   Williams

Nicole Payen, Clymenza Hawkins, Michelle Williams, and
   Kellie Jones, Ph.D.(iva)

Erica Simone Turnipseed, Lynn Nottage, and Tonya Meeks

Dawne Simon-Ponte, Linda Heppard, and Elizabeth Hunte

Cassandra Hughes Webster and McKenzii Denise Webster

Sally Hensley, Austin Jennings, Anthony Williams, Dolores
   Digaetano, and Marva Souder

Friday Afternoon Tea in Cooper-Young; Memphis, Tennessee,
   Midtown Yoga

Sarla, Jimmy, Arline, Leah, and the entire crew


And, of course, Derek Bonner

# contents

**Five**

**Six**

**Seven**

**Eight**

**Nine**

**Ten**

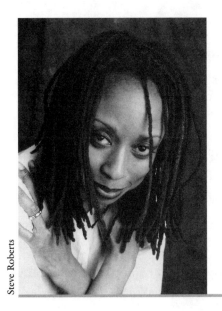

Steve Roberts

ThankYou for Letting Me Be Myself . . . Again

When I decided to lock my hair, a gift to myself in the prime of my life, I figured that the growing of my locks and the wearing of them would be fairly straightforward. After all, I'd written two hair memoirs—*Good Hair: For Colored Girls Who've Considered Weaves When the Chemicals Became Too Ruff* and *Plaited Glory: For Colored Girls Who've Considered Braids Locks and Twists,* and I believed I was respectably familiar with the Commandments of Locking One's Hair:

- Your hair must be nappy.
- You must cut off your perm.
- If you don't want to cut off your perm you can grow it out with braids.
- Beeswax makes your locks look good.
- Don't wash your hair for three months.
- Stock up on a supply of scarves that you can wear around your hairline while your hair is locking. Better yet, dust off your hat collection.
- Grit your teeth and square your shoulders through the buckwheat stage.
- Keep your locks twisted.
- Don't let them get too dry.

So, what was the problem?

The problem was that I wanted Nice Dreads. I wanted people to say, "She's got Nice Dreads." That was very important to me. In Memphis, Tennessee, having Nice Hair is very important. In Memphis, dreads are not Nice Hair, so it was important that I have Nice Dreads if I were to have any at all. I didn't really think that the Niceness would win over the Memphis Nap Patrol but I imagined that it would allow me to slide under the radar without overt criticism, cloaked in protective Niceness.

Still, I fretted. Maybe I wouldn't be as lovable with

locks. Maybe it was true, the naps wouldn't be as pretty as my miracle hair, my trademark corkscrew twist-outs, the ones I'd waxed so poetically about in *Good Hair*, the two-strand twists that when unfurled left my hair in a bush of wildly glorious nappy corkscrews that strangers admired and wanted for themselves. The twists I'd doctored with a little chemical texturizer. Some so-called "hair purists" had tried to dismiss my contribution to hair diversity as not being "natural." These were the same purists who saw nothing unnatural about braiding Asian hair extensions into "natural" hair. I'd held tough; I wasn't chemical free, but I had them on a technicality because my hair wasn't straightened. The distinction I made was promoting an aesthetic that worked with coily hair, not against it. I'd had a good run with my twists and now maybe I was playing fast and loose with a good hair thing. Maybe people wouldn't praise my hair anymore; after all, these were dreadlocks. I was wading in high water, no turning back.

I have admired locks ever since I first saw them in the early 1980s on the late actress Rosalind Cash. I'd been attending a Dance Theatre of Harlem performance in Pasadena, California. Being a clothing maven, I was impressed first with Ms. Cash's full-length mink coat—and then I noticed her hair. It appeared to be in a halo of coils that was mid-length between her chin and shoulders. I had no idea what style it was. I knew it wasn't an afro; it was more like a free-form bush studded with twists and coils. I made inquiries and discovered that Ms. Cash was wearing her hair in what they called *dreadlocks*. I remember seeing another African American actress at the same event; she had recently appeared in *Playboy* and wore her hair in a straightened, shoulder-length pageboy that moved in the breeze. Until then, seeing a glamorous starlet up close with the fabled blow-hair I'd coveted and chased for years would have been a "beautiful people" moment, but that night it left me cold. It was Ms. Cash and her wild locks who made the biggest impression on me.

Now I won't lie and say that I was into Rastafarian dreadlocks from way back; back then, I didn't have the cultural sophistication to appreciate them. I related more to attractive women who wore cultivated locks. I'd gaze at their hair hungrily, how it flowed down their backs, the best part being that it was all their own. Women who were starting their locks, the coily nappy buds crowning their heads, had a smug confidence about them because they knew that it was only a matter of time before their hair would sprout into locks that would make their way past their shoulders and beyond. I noticed the different textures, how tighter hair spun itself into felted locks and softer hair spun into locks of an intertwined randomness. I coveted the heaviness of wearing locked hair in a sexy, messy topknot. I admired the hair of locked artists—Cassandra Wilson, Rosalind Cash, Whoopi Goldberg, Alice Walker, Angela Davis, Vanessa L. Williams, India.Arie, Tracie Chapman, Lisa Bonet, Bethann Hardison, Suzan-Lori Parks, Toni Morrison. I was delighted to read a wonderful essay written by Anne Lamott, a white writer whose lifelong struggle to wrestle her beautiful, tightly coiled hair into straight acceptance had been the bane of her beauty existence. Then, one fine day, after Ms. Lamott declared she was indeed ready, a locked sister took her in hand and started Ms. Lamott's locks. Now, she peers out at the world from behind her locks "as through a beautiful handmade fence, in the drizzle, in the wind, in the rain." I heard that.

I was surprised and flattered when people in Memphis asked if my corkscrew twists were dreadlocks. Finally, it boiled down to my lust for locks and a desire to make myself happy for the rest of my life. What the heck; these people think I'm wearing locks anyway and I'm not even enjoying the benefits. Why not go for the gusto?

When I decided to lock my hair, I believed I could fashion a new way to dread, that I could retain the shiny gloss that comes with baby coils, that my locks, due to my genetic gift of soft hair, would look like nappy Shirley Temple curls. This is also known as a *straw set*. The texture of the hair on the crown of my head is more loosely coiled than the hair at my temples and back; the hair at my nape, known in African American culture as *the kitchen,* is soft and springy. In short, different degrees of coil, but in plain language, nappy all the same.

I began by softening my hair with water until it clumped into coils. I'd been growing it out from a texturizer for a few months, and it was about five inches long with about two inches of springy new growth. The texturized hair was slightly looser and retained a slightly loosened coil at the end. This, I believed, would make locking no problem, as the ends weren't bone straight and my locks would look pretty if they ended in coily curled tips.

Parting my hair into sections a little smaller than the circumference of a pencil, I applied a dab of chocolate brown Pre Con gel to each section and rolled it between my palms until it resembled a long coil of straw set hair. It took about two hours to do my entire head in this manner, and the result, I thought, gave me a baby coil look with lots of shine. I had visible partings on my scalp—not a look I considered flattering—but the gel had encouraged the hair closest to the scalp to wave and smoothed down the unruly halo around my hairline, so I considered myself extremely presentable. Translation: Nice Dreads. Good Locks. Once the locks took hold, I could show the world it was indeed possible to start locks without negotiating one's way through the Buckwheat stage. After all, I was a Hair Diva, author of three books; I had to *represent*.

Now water does a lot of things to the hair shaft: It makes it pliable; it opens the tiny shingles that coat the shaft so conditioners can penetrate; it makes the hair revert to its natural tendency to wave, curl, or lie straight. Water encourages the coils in curly hair to group together into larger coils instead of separating into frizz. Add enough gel, and you can coax a wave out of hair as tight as a watch spring. But applying water and gel does not change the texture of the hair one is genetically programmed to grow nor does it change the texture of hair that has been chemically altered. These laws of hair nature had flown out of my head, for when my hair dried, I noticed that the bulk of the coils I'd painstakingly shellacked and palm-rolled into place had puffed into nappy stogies with the texture and density of cotton candy.

Only the chemically free hair, the three or so inches of hair near the root, maintained splendid and glossy coils that were smooth against my fingertips.

All the blathering I'd done in print about cutting off processed hair for the good of the rest of the hair echoed in my head, bounced off the bathroom walls. It was like performing euthanasia on a beloved pet who was suffering; I

knew what needed to be done, yet I just couldn't bring myself to do it. But when I looked in the mirror, I knew I had
to put on my game face and find a loctician. For the unini-
tiated, a loctician is a person who grooms and styles locks.

I was afraid I'd be busted out for having a texturizer in
my hair, that I would walk into the salon and be told in no
uncertain terms that my ends would have to go, that I'd
hang my head shamefaced.

My high-handed attitude toward Memphis hair trends
notwithstanding, I reasoned that someone who could twist
up pipe-cleaner-tight coils for the sporting men around
town could lay a foundation for my locks. I asked around,
and the name that came up more than once was Nefertiti
(not her real name), so off I went to see the wizard. She
was renting from a communal shop in the community with
the usual accoutrements: no children or food allowed in the
shop, no receptionist, toilet paper on ration in the bath-
rooms—these were temporary accommodations, as she was
setting up to open her own location soon. Meanwhile, it
gave me ghetto salon flashbacks. It felt like home.

Nefertiti's locks were a thick raven black, spun into locks
the circumference of pipe cleaners. They were curled into a
mass of ringlets that cascaded down her shoulders. Good
advertising for the lock hungry. Lord knew how much

maintenance went into grooming locks of that size and abundance. I clearly had no idea. But she was a loctician with a fierce-looking head of locks, and I was hungry.

I came clean, spit out the truth—that I was growing out a texturizer—and braced myself.

Nefertiti looked at me over the line of heads waiting to be done and read me like an old issue of *People* magazine.

"No, you don't have to cut off your perm."

I took my place at the shampoo bowl.

Nefertiti's hook was Locks Without Busting Your Chops, and I grabbed it like a Jheri Curl holdout snatching the last bottle of activator at the beauty supply shop.

First, she washed my scalp with a coal tar shampoo to lift the flakes. I hadn't had a coal tar shampoo since childhood. Coal tar is an old school remedy for dandruff. It felt good, and I reasoned that a flaky scalp wasn't the greatest foundation for a set of locks. After the shampoo, I took my place in the lineup.

A Nefertiti client was sitting next to me; her hair, in locks the size of Nefertiti's, was up in rollers. I had a hair talk with her and she testified about the sanctity of locks. I hung on to every word. Her hair was thick, with no scalp showing. Nefertiti's style was to spin small locks that could be curled and styled like straight hair. My aesthetic leaned toward allowing locks to hang loose and free rather than curling them, but once I was locked, I could wear them any way I wanted.

I hopped into Nefertiti's chair. My "locks"—the twisted stogies with the coiled roots—had survived the shampoo. I told her I was seeking a shape-up, just a little push to get my locks into shape. She told me that because of the texture or *textures* of my hair, two-strand twists were the best way to start my locks.

"No problem," she said, and commenced oiling, gelling, and retwisting. Each retwisted lock was secured with a metal clip. The locks were looking mighty tight and shiny, with plenty of scalp showing—a look I would wear in the privacy of my own home, not one I relished going into public with. She explained that small locks were best for my hair because if she made them larger, it was possible that as my hair grew, the lock would become too heavy, put stress on the roots, and pull my hair out. "Think of the horror of losing locks that way after two or three years of growing," she said. "They thicken up and fill in as they mature." I kept taking looks at her locks whenever I could crane my head around to do so; they were thin and she surely had a head full of them. I was sold.

She put me under the dryer and was on to the next head. The dryer set my twists—really couldn't call them locks just yet. I looked, as they say, mighty new.

"You need to come back every two weeks for washing and retwisting until they start to lock," she said. It was forty dollars a pop, easy on my budget.

A couple weeks into my new lock-twists, I paid a visit to my family. The Memphis branch of my family had always been rather conservative when it comes to hair, but the elders had somewhat tolerated afros and cornrows back in the day. However, just as soon as they'd praised the Lord that those days were over, here came the second wave, the cornrows, freedom hair, afros, twists, braids, Nubian knots, and coils—but the worst of the lot, hands down, were dreadlocks. By then, my family pretty much knew that I "went my own way," the nappy way. I was determined to practice some of what I'd preached.

"Those look like the twists you do yourself," said my cousin.

Yeah, but I wanted to start them off right, I said, get the partings even, because this is the foundation, the grid for my locks.

*"Dreadlocks?"* she asked.

"Yep, I'm locking," I said.

"What if you want to take them out?" asked another cousin.

You can't take them out once they're locked, I replied.

"You have to cut your hair to get them out?"

Yep. I waited to lock because I wanted to be sure, I replied.

They gave me that "I guess you know what you're doing" look. Frankly, I knew I was just about to strike out. Strike One: Dreadlocks! Strike Two: You couldn't take them out unless you cut off your hair.

"What does Derek think?" they asked. Derek is my husband.

"He likes them, he likes my hair. He wants me to let them grow really long," I said.

"Well, Lonnice is lucky because Derek likes them but *all* men don't *like* dreadlocks." Strike Three.

If I was headed for the dugout, I was going out with dignity. I wasn't going to throw the bat.

"Well, sure, everyone has their tastes," I said, "but if you're wearing locks and looking good, what's not to like?" Plus, I knew that my cousin had been a hair rebel in Memphis, sporting an afro and cornrows back in the day. I had begged my mother to let me have cornrows like hers, and my mother had given me the thumbs down. I think my cousin was secretly down with the program, but she had to be a mom. After all, Memphis is not on the cutting edge of Afrocentric hair culture. When I moved to Memphis in 1998, I noticed folks who still wore plastic shower caps during the week so their Jheri Curls would be fresh on the weekend.

I never got an opportunity to play with some other members of my family. I knew my elders weren't into naps, and whatever they really thought of my hair was best left unsaid or said when I was out of the room. Still, I received acknowledgment from my other cousins, who would check out how consistently my locked hair grew.

"Girl, they're going to start calling you Rapunzel!"

Meanwhile, a couple weeks after my visit to Nefertiti's, I noticed that my lock-twists hadn't begun to swell and fill in the partings on my scalp. I shampooed them before my next appointment—surely I knew more than a little about locks, I thought—but they didn't hide my scalp. I locked myself in the bathroom, took out each of the twists Nefertiti had put in, and made each parting smaller, doubling the number of twists in my hair. The increase in the number of twists didn't make my hair look any fuller. I just had a lot more small twists on my head. The ends looked spindly.

I went back to Nefertiti for my coal tar shampoo and retwist and mentioned I'd made them smaller. She assured me that as the twists locked, I would get the fullness I craved. I clung to that hope.

Each day I'd examine my lock-twists, faithfully tying them down at night, maintaining the tightened roots, wanting to ensure that my locks were even. Aware that one stray nap would throw me out of the running for Nice

Dreads, I monitored the roots and kept them tight. Much too tight. I was one twisted sister.

I'd been invited to the New York premiere and party for a cable feature my dear friend Lisa had written. Unfortunately, my locks were not what I'd hoped they'd be. Suddenly it was important to me that they look like locks, whether they were nappy or whatever. The hair limbo I was caught up in was beginning to drive me to distraction.

So, when I got to the city, Lisa called some locked friends of hers and got some recommendations on lock salons. I chose Khamit Kinks, in SoHo. That's where I turned the corner and began to lock, thanks to Doc, the Loc Doctor.

My girl Lisa accompanied me to my appointment with Doc for a hot oil treatment and lock grooming session that was scheduled to last for about an hour. Poor Lisa waited as I ended up spending five hours in Doc's chair, no extra charge, simply because he took pride in his work and could see that my hair needed the correction. It was worth every minute.

He went by the name Doc because his special talent was being a lock doctor, getting locks into shape. He was an honest young man, and he gave it to me straight. What he told me was this: Maybe not now, not tomorrow, next week, or even next month, but know that the perm is going to go. It can go out with dignity, a clean cut and a fresh start. Or it can go out like a punk, thin and broken rat-tail ends hanging, the two textures fighting against each other. No one wins here except the Nap Patrol, because they are vindicated.

"See," they could say, "those dreads look like crap," and here you are in the flesh proving their every word. For the first time, I saw the light, and it wasn't pretty. It was the Nappy Horror Picture Show.

SEE the pepper balls at the nape of her neck!

HEAR the sound of fingernails clawing at a scalp that hasn't been washed in a month of Sundays!

WATCH her try to hide her hair under a head wrap!

KNOW that even the oldest played-out perm looks better than that nappy mess!

All I had to do was let him do his job. I sat in his chair and watched women and men come in and get their locks and braids hooked up. He coached me as he worked on my hair. "Don't twist so much," he said. "Let your hair do what it does. Just keep them separated. It will be okay. You've got to get used to your hair again. I'm putting some of these twists together because they're too small and they're not going to make it. I'm trimming you up to the good hair—the nappy hair—and a month from now, you're gonna see the difference. Try not to wash it for two weeks but after then you should be okay. You've heard of Dr. Bronner's liquid soap? Use that; it's the best. If any locks come loose when you wash your hair, just retwist them. I know it looks tight, but you'll be thanking me in about six weeks.

"You probably won't have to see me again," he said.

Those were words I'd never before heard a hairdresser, loctician, or cosmetologist say, and I haven't heard them since. They turned out to be true. I didn't and don't have to see him again, but believe me, anyone who does you a good turn definitely has your loyalty and your future business.

A month later, my hair had begun to look as if it were truly locking. It all boiled down to creating the proper foundation that allowed my hair to do what it does best. The baggage in my mind was like weeds in my garden. When I chucked them, my hair began to flourish.

# One

# Getting Started: Fruit of the Nappy Root

The main things folks want to know about starting locks are (1) Do I have to cut off my perm? and (2) Can you take them out?

First things first. Black women and haircuts have a stormy history. There's a natural distrust of cutting, trimming, or putting any sort of sharp edge to our hair. I believe this is because we've been misled for so long about the fabled benefits of cutting that we're just naturally wary.

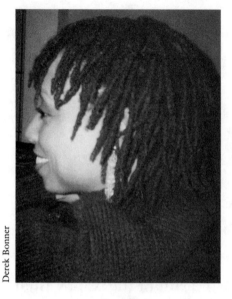

Derek Bonner

This picture was taken on Christmas 2001. My locks are a year old, and it's the first time they actually began to look like locks. Two months before, when Doc cut off my raggedy, processed ends, he told me that this would be my reward.

We're trying to keep some hair, grow some hair, but when we go to the hairdresser we always end up giving them some. That's because we swallow the correlation between touch-ups and trims; your new growth needs a touch-up and you trim the ends. Some hairdressers will throw game instead of skills and tell you that you need the trim because it will make your hair stronger, help it grow. What actually happens is that they trim whatever you grow so your hair remains in stasis. If your hair is overprocessed—a chronic condition in Black hair care—you'll have chronic breakage, which guarantees you'll never really see any meaningful increase in length. The trim is simply a cosmetic stave-off that keeps your hair presentable and makes their work look good when you leave the chair.

Another factor is fear of the unknown. We know how our perm is going to work; we're accustomed to managing our expectations when it comes to touch-ups, breakage, and making nappy hair straight. All the energy has been directed toward achieving and maintaining straightness. The very idea of long lush hair that comes from the nappy coils we've been taught to remove is, well, an idea that takes many women some time to get used to.

I believe many Black women experience a visual oxymoron when they see long locked hair. It can't be real because everyone knows that nappy hair doesn't grow long enough to hang, it only grows out, as in an afro. Plus, the long hair fantasy—Rapunzel, Indian-Runs-in-My-Family, Goldilocks, Cher, Darchelle on Solid Gold, Jan and Marcia, the Asian Chick on Soul Train when Don Cornelius was the host—is all about long, *straight* hair or braid extensions tricked up to look like straight hair. Not dreadlocks. So when women see waist-length locks they see a comb and a dream; if they can comb it out and make it straight, they can get to the Promised Land.

I wish somebody had taken me in hand and told me to focus on what was important and forget the nonsense. The questions you should be asking when you are thinking about locking your hair should revolve around starting techniques and how you can expect your locks to look in the early weeks and months. You should know something about various locking methods, much as you would inquire about how to cultivate flowers you have never grown before. If you keep that analogy in mind, the ridiculous concern about whether or not you have to cut off your perm—or cut your hair, period—will make about as much sense as asking if you need to get rid of the concrete before you can plant a garden in the same spot.

## DO I HAVE TO CUT OFF MY PERM?

The short answer is yes, but you'll never look back in regret unless you weren't really ready to go for it in the first place. If you want strong, aesthetically appealing locks, the perm just has to go.

## CAN YOU TAKE LOCKS OUT?

I assume those who want to know how to do this remain deliriously excited about the possibility that waist-length locks can mean waist-length unlocked hair. I will categorically state that should you have the tenacity to pick apart an entire head of locks, you will not retain anything near the length of your locked hair. Get a grip and get yourself some braid extensions, which can be removed periodically with the goal of retaining the growth and length of your own hair. You'll be happier.

## ANATOMY OF A LOCK

Locked hair is a coily paradox. In order to form locks that flow down straight, the coils must be allowed to mesh and intertwine, encouraged to spin together into a cylindrical shaft of hair. Individual coiled strands grow and rest during the hair's life cycle. When the hair is shed, the released coil remains intertwined in the lock. The unlocked hair at the base is alive and growing from the hair follicles; the body of each lock is akin to a large shaft of hair.

The average growth rate of hair is about one half-inch per month. Remember that this is an average rate; some hair grows faster or slower, and factors like age, health, pregnancy, and heredity have different effects on your hair's growth rate.

Human hair grows in three stages. In the *catogen* stage, the hair prepares to emerge from the follicle. The growth phase, which can last from two to six years, is called the *anogen* stage. The resting stage, called the *telogen* stage, lasts for about three months, and then the hair is shed. Hair tends to grow faster in warm seasons than in colder ones.

The longer your hair's anogen phase lasts, the more predisposed you are to have longer hair. For example, it takes about six years to grow waist-length hair from a short haircut, given a growth or anogen phase of at least six years. It's fairly clear that women with waist-length hair have some genetic advantage going for them, but plenty of women have hair flowing pretty close to that length. How is this possible?

Well, in many cases, it isn't so much about hair growth as it is about *retention* of that growth—it simply means that women with long, beautiful hair are working their program consistently. Those of us of African descent should also remember that tightly coiled hair tends to appear shorter, often half the length of straight hair of the same length. However, when these same strands intertwine and spin around each other, the hair is contained in cylindrical units and the ends are amazingly protected, and the hair, clean and conditioned, is retained along with the shed hair, spun into a lock like the finest of soft yarns.

It is helpful to compare the stages of lock development to those of the stages of individual hair strand growth, with sprouting, growing, resting, and shedding stages.

Five stages mark the process of your hair as the coils intertwine and spin themselves into cylindrical locks:

1. **Coils**—Coils resemble tightly coiled springs that look like baby spirals and can be as small as a watch spring or fluid and loose as fusilli. Hair can be as short or as long as one likes. The key factor here is that your hair is able to form and hold a coil, but the hair within the coil has not yet begun to intertwine or mesh.

What people find attractive about coils is that the hair tends to have sheen or shine because of the light that re-fracts off of the bend in each tiny ringlet. This is the first ex-perience many African American women with extremely coily hair have with hair that naturally shines, without oiling or greasing. Coils work like bait, because often a woman sees another woman with a head full of coils and begins to consider the possibilities.

2. **Sprouts and Buds**—Crudely known among the philistines as Knots and Peas, Buckwheat Stage, Pickaninny Stage, Nappy Stage, "I wish she'd take that out" stage. Among the enlightened, initiated, erudite, urban hip chic set, cultural BAPs, and so on, your hair is recognized as Sprouting or Budding in that miraculous moment when the magic has begun. Those who are mothers can liken this to the terrible twos; it can be a challenging and creative time, or you can pull your hair out in frustration and give up. Would you give up your child because he was a terrible

two? Naw, you just work with it and through it because you understand that what you do at this time sets the stage for the rest of his childhood development. The idea is to let him have his space while still setting boundaries, because trying to apply too much reason with a toddler is—well, you get the picture. Now apply that analogy to your sprouting and budding locks.

First, you shampoo your hair and notice that all of a sudden, the coils don't all wash out like they used to. You may notice that some of your coils have little knots of hair in them, about the size of a small pea. This knot is more or less the nucleus of each lock; the hairs in your coils have begun to intertwine and interlace. Individual coils may seem puffy and lose their tightly coiled shape; this is part of the process and shouldn't be disturbed. What is important here is to keep the original scalp partings, to allow the spinning process to become established for each individual lock. Don't redivide your budding locks, twist them to death, or get to patting them down, trying to make your hair look "nice," because you'll just end up with a badly packed, busted-out do that is neither fish nor 'fro. You'll look like you're ashamed and embarrassed, and your hair will look downright bad because you'll be cowering from it, walking around like hey, this isn't me, this isn't my hair. Lord, it sure is nappy. Don't mind me,

I'm on my way to get a relaxer. Oops! You caught me before I put my wig on this morning. And the anti-nap people will be on you like a duck on a junebug.

As I explained, buds are pea-shaped bubbles of hair that form either at the end of a small lock or in the middle of the budding lock. The bud is the nucleus of the intertwining transformation of hair. Sometimes buds become detached from the individual lock; these can be removed. Detached buds are little balls of hair that hang off the tips of some locks, suspended by a strand or two of hair. As long as the bud of hair is firmly meshed and attached to the rest of the lock, it is progressing fine. Some folks enjoy the funky, edgy look of wild little spirals and coils; others desperately want to avoid the Buckwheat phase.

Many women discover that indeed their hair has a coily texture and they're now the closest they've ever been to having a true natural curl—albeit tight and tiny, but curls nonetheless. Budding can be a time when you learn a lot about your hair and have a good time with it as it grows into shoots, or you can go against the grain and be miserable and embarrassed because your hair is nappy. I received plenty of kudos from strangers during this phase. Some recognized that I was locking my hair; others didn't know what I was doing with my hair, but they liked it.

3. **Teen or Locking Stage**—This is when the buds and sprouts truly begin to look like locks and few, if any, locks shampoo out or come out during sleep. The peas you saw and felt in the budding stage have expanded, and the hair has spun into a network of intertwining strands that extend throughout the length of individual locks. The locks may be soft and pliable or feel loosely meshed, according to your hair's texture. This is the anogen or growing stage of lock development, and it extends into the lock's mature stage. Shampooing doesn't loosen these locks. They have dropped, which means they have developed enough to hang down versus defying gravity. This is when you start to relax and feel more confident about locking.

4. **Mature Stage**—Each individual lock is firmly meshed or tightly interwoven. Some loosely coiled hair textures may retain a small curl or coil at the end of the locks, but most will probably be closed at the ends. You will begin to see consistent growth because each lock has intertwined and contracted into a cylindrical shape. Think of each individual lock as a hair strand in itself. The new growth is contained in the loose hair at the base or root of each individual lock, and regular grooming encourages it to spin into an intertwined coil that will be integrated with the lock.

5. **Beyond Maturity**—Think of this stage as akin to the shedding stage of hair growth. After many years, depending on the care you have lavished on your locks, some locks may begin to thin and break off at the ends. For the most part, this deterioration can be minimized and controlled by monitoring the ends of your locks for signs of age and getting regular trims.

Remember, these are simply guidelines to development, not hair length. In fact, until your locks are mature, it is much better that you pay attention to the stages of development rather than length because any length you attain before the locks mature is likely to change or shorten as you continue to spin and groom your locks and the strands intertwine and contract into cylinders.

My preoccupation with length during my first year of locking caused me to hang on to my few inches of texturized hair and probably slowed the locking process. Hair hunger blinded me to the limp rat-tail twists trailing the plump budding locks. Sitting in Khamit Kinks loctician Doc's chair and listening to him explain the futility of keeping two or three inches of old, played-out hair that only served to make my locks look raggedy was my salvation. The texturized, processed hair did not coil up with the virgin hair, and it never would. Sure, no one likes to hear that after getting through the buds and sprouts you're going to be taken back to that length, but the overall look was such an aesthetic improvement that I didn't miss the length at all. After the cutting my locks were even, they were tight, and just like Doc said, three months—heck, eight weeks—later, they rocked.

## GETTING STARTED

Spin your coils into manicured locks or let them free-form into a felted crown. It's your style; it's your call. For a cultivated look, begin by parting the hair into sections, the same as when parting for individual braids. The idea is to establish a grid or foundation for your locks. Each sectioned lock is cultivated or manicured by regular palm rolling or twisting. Free-form or Rasta locks are locks that are allowed to form in a random pattern, but they are still maintained by palm rolling or twisting. Contrary to popular belief, free-formed locks are not any less clean than manicured or cultivated locks; they are simply a variation in style and appearance. For instance, a cultural BAP might be down with a nicely groomed free-form, while her boho sister rocks ultramanicured, perfectly uniform WASP locks. The appearance of locks depends on your hereditary curl pattern.

Let's clear up some lock mythology. Folks get to whispering about beeswax, lemon juice, beer and vinegar rinses, glue—whatever. If your natural hair texture is nappy, you don't need any of that stuff.

When I scout the shelves of beauty supply stores, I notice pure beeswax being touted as a locking aid. Beeswax is a crutch that has traditionally been used to help get hair through the budding stage without retwisting and grooming after a shampoo. Because it is a water repellent, beeswax is difficult to shampoo from the hair and will build up on your locks. Petrolatum, used as a cheap filler in hairdressings, also repels water and will coat your locks. Some beeswax products for locking hair contain petrolatum as well. These products coat the hair with a barrier that doesn't allow penetration of oils and moisturizers; this will eventually dry out your locks. I don't recommend beeswax because it is so difficult to remove and is unnecessary for hair locking.

If you're a Rainbow baby with hair that is naturally straight or loosely waved, you should understand that locking may be difficult for you, and people do use wax and glue to make it work. Locking these textures is like making extremely coiled hair bone straight—it can be done, but it won't be easy, and sometimes it may be more trouble than the hair can stand. However, our Caucasian brothers and sisters lock their hair and the look is more like matting than actual coiling. Still, I respect and share their admiration for the coil; imitation is the sincerest form of flattery.

## The Hookup

The ideal situation is to have a loctician or braider start your locks for you. Your best bet is a loctician, a stylist who specializes in starting, grooming, and styling locks. You can find a loctician in the same way you would sniff out any other Afrocentric stylist; ask around, ask locked women who does their hair. What you are looking for is someone with skills who can lay down a grid for your locks. You can arrange a session to start off your locks and follow the loctician's instructions on how to maintain them. Do be aware that this is a business and respect the fact that locticians have to eat like everyone else, but don't be sucked into a "see me every week" game just like the one you thought you'd escaped with the perm. Unless this sort of thing is what you want.

If you have any weak moments in deciding about whether or not to lock your hair, a visit to a *good* loctician can boost your confidence while offering a reality check. Locticians can give you positive reinforcement about wearing and caring for locks. Any loctician worth his salt will have a fierce head of locks by example, which can only spur you on. You'll meet other locked heads, and you can share locking tales and grooming tips. If you have a hair texture that's hard to lock, then a loctician is certainly a good idea because he can tell you what you can (or cannot) expect. You can, of course, start and groom your own locks, but if possible, get a friend to help with the initial partings (unless you intend to free-form) so your locks will be evenly distributed and formed.

## What You'll Need to Begin

- **Water** in a spray bottle for dampening your hair and encouraging it to coil. You can also use leave-in conditioner in spray formula or make your own herbal infusion. Many locticians have their own formulas. You can try ¼ cup dried rosemary and ¼ cup dried nettle steeped in 4 cups of water. If you use fresh herbs, increase each portion of herbs to ½ cup. You can buy the dried herbs at health food stores and find fresh rosemary in the supermarket produce section.

- **Hair clips** to separate your hair into sections.

- A **mirror** so you can see what you're doing.

- A **holding agent** like a locking gel or aloe vera. The idea is to help hold the hair in position until it stays put. A water-soluble holding agent can be washed away easily without leaving a sticky film, which is why, in comparison, beeswax is a bad idea. Beeswax might get you started, but you will be hard-pressed to get it out of your hair—and you will want to when your buds are gray with old beeswax buildup.

**Optional But Nice**
- A **bonnet-style hair dryer** will help set your freshly twisted hair, but you can certainly let your locks dry naturally. Allowing your locks to dry naturally is a good habit to establish.

## Locking Short Hair

### FREE-FORM

If you like free-form locks, then you can start with the Rasta method, where you allow your locks to bud randomly and then maintain whatever size and shape they lock into.

### BRAIDS

This method is probably most appropriate for hair textures that are extremely soft and resistant to locking. With this shortcut, you won't have that attractive cylindrical look that comes from the traditional coiling methods. Part your hair in sections about the width of your finger and braid each section into a small plait. If your hair is very loosely curled, you can apply styling gel to help hold the plait together. You will have a plaited look at the end of your locks for a year or more until the lock matures.

## Locking Hair That's Midlength or Longer

### PALM ROLLING

Starting from the nape of your neck, take sections of the hair about the width of a finger. Take smaller sections of the delicate nape hair so the locks can grow long without placing stress on the hairline. Dampen the hair with water or leave-in conditioner. If your hair responds to gel, use a bit of that. Roll the section between your palms in one direction, encouraging the hair to roll into a cylindrical coil or spiral.

### TWO-STRAND TWISTS

This is the method I used to start my locks. I was impatient and wanted my locks to look like locked hair. Looking back, the transition was efficient and fast, and I love the way my locks turned out. Starting at the nape of your neck, take sections of your hair that are about the width of a pencil or your finger. Dampen the section with water and/or your holding agent and separate it into two strands. Twist the strands together into a braid. The ends will coil around one another, but if they want to unfurl, give them a spritz of water and retwist them.

## Extra-Small Locks

Small or skinny locks require more maintenance than larger locks. The general rule is the circumference of a pencil or your finger. Remember that the smaller the lock, the more delicate it will be and the more maintenance it will require. Smaller locks break more easily. The exception is the locks you spin along your hairline where the hair is softer and less tolerant of tension. It's nice to have thinner locks around your temples and hairline that can frame your face.

If you want super-small locks, then the method known as Sisterlocks would be better for you. This locking technique, developed by Dr. Joanne Cornwell, requires a special tool to lock the hair. Sisterlocks must be put in by a trained consultant, and in order to tighten your own locks you must take a class taught by a certified Sisterlocks consultant. (See Resources, page 142, for the Sisterlocks web address.) Do know going into this method that maintenance is extremely important, as the individual locks are so small that they will indeed mat at the scalp if you are not diligent about regular tightening.

Keep in mind that extremely small micro-locks require

the assistance of a professional loctician. Those spaghetti-thin locks can be striking and versatile, but as the old folks say, "If you give a dance, you gotta pay the band."

## ADJUSTING TO YOUR NEW LOOK

Some days your hair will be really cute. Other days, it will need a little help. Here are a few suggestions to help you through the transitions.

- Hair isn't cooperating today? Wrap a pretty scarf around your hairline and let the coils frame the scarf.
- Don't pack your hair down in an effort to make it look less Buckwheatish. It's okay to finger-shape your hair into a halo, but packing crushes your budding locks and looks unflattering.
- Keep your buds and shoots twisted, but don't over do it. Reread the section on the stages of locking and remind yourself not to stifle your hair's development.
- Keep your hair lubricated; supple hair encourages the natural coil formation that is essential to the locking process.
- Meet other women who wear locks. Go on the Internet. Buy hair magazines that feature locked hair. Feed your mind.

- Don't become discouraged and get lazy about keeping up with your locks. Remember that the beginning stages are temporary and will soon pass. Maintenance is key!

## STAYING STRONG, STAYING LOCKED

You will attract some attention when you are locking your hair. Many women have told me that when they began locking their hair, they were complimented at a rate that seldom occurred when their hair was straightened. Sometimes strangers will want to touch your hair. It can get tiresome being a hair ambassador, but look at it this way—they could be throwing eggs. I don't recommend letting strangers touch you or your hair. You can usually tell the difference between someone who is crowding your space and someone who is genuinely interested in locking her hair. Try to keep a sense of humor about it, but be careful.

## Two

### How Do You *Wash* Them?

"*Can* you wash them?"

"They look so *clean*."

"How do you keep them so *clean*?"

"Tell Daddy how you wash them."

Somehow, the tallest, thorniest hurdle those who aspire to wear locks must clear is the issue of cleanliness. The crux of the issue is this: I was afraid to look as if I'd slept in a box on the street. Hair matted into a street pillow against my head, nasty, unclean. Some might wonder why I would even care about what some philistines thought about my do.

"You've written three books about nappy hair." Big deal.

"You've been on *Oprah*!" So what.

"Your hair is (gonna be) down to your waist!"

Well, this is one case in the history of a people who have done everything possible to buy, weave, sew, glue, plant, pray, and marry themselves into some good hair where long hair doesn't mean doo-doo. "You mean, you'd rather see me with a head full of Korean Yakky hair treated to look like it was nappy straightened hair, bonded or sewed into my hair, than a head of my own hair, beautifully groomed locks hanging past my waist?" In many circles in the South, the answer is "Yes, indeedy!"

You see, the case against nappiness is one strike, but the Nap Patrol's spitball combination of declaring that "Your hair looks nasty" is often too much for all but the hardiest lock novice to overcome. This is because of the longstanding taboo against nastiness. In African American culture, "nasty" has a certain distinction. A woman is not called nasty because she snaps at a grocery clerk. Please don't make the mistake of confusing dirtiness with nastiness, because as far as the African American community is concerned, being dirty is far more acceptable than being nasty.

Dirt can be washed away. Nastiness is a condition, a lifestyle.

All it takes is a simple declaration, delivered in a character slamming sotto voce through clenched teeth, punctuated by a raised eyebrow and cocked head—"You *know*, she's *nasty*."—to guarantee that no one will touch your spinach and crab dip at the housewarming. Then someone whispers this social roundhouse: "Her house *stays* nasty." A "nasty house" tag can taint your children's neighborhood rating until they are grown and have their own houses and even then, the old folks will keep the memory alive, expecting the worst, because they knew your mother kept a nasty house . . . bless her heart.

Alice Walker wrote *Essence* magazine in the 1990s about its comments concerning locks and the unwashed. Her letter cited a reference to not shampooing the hair for three months. She took exception to the comment and felt compelled to write because, as she so rightly pointed out, one of the enticements of locks is the freedom to wash one's hair as frequently as one likes without worrying about ruining a hairstyle or having the hair revert if it has been straightened. She feared readers would take this faulty information to heart and feel that three months of "dirty" hair was too high a price to pay for the eventual freedom of locks—and who could blame them? Amen.

## OKAY, ENOUGH ALREADY! HOW OFTEN SHOULD I WASH MY LOCKS?

You should shampoo your hair when your scalp feels dirty. When perspiration mixes with the natural shedding of the scalp and dirty sebum, it's time to hit the water. When the scalp oils or sebum are incorporated with dirt and other effluvia, the smell is not pretty. This matter piles up and, if it is not removed, becomes embedded in the intertwining coils of each lock. At this point you will notice grayish matter around the base of each lock. This matter, along with bad choices in grooming products like beeswax and conditioners that don't completely rinse out, is the core ingredient of buildup. Buildup is hard to remove. Buildup attracts extra lint. Buildup gives your locks a grayish tinge. Buildup wreaks havoc when you try to color your hair.

You can temporarily refresh your scalp with a dry shampoo. You'll need gauze, which comes in both rolls and squares, or a generous piece of cheesecloth. Take a piece of cheesecloth or gauze and wrap it around your index finger. The cheesecloth can be used dry or moistened with Sea Breeze or witch hazel. Part the hair so as to expose the scalp partings for each lock and rub the scalp in a gently brisk massaging motion. Change the piece of the gauze or cheesecloth at intervals when it becomes soiled; a refresher won't be effective if you are trying to clean your scalp with a grimy piece of cloth. When the entire scalp is cleaned in this way, you get the dual benefit of cleanliness and the stimulation that encourages hair growth.

The scalp refresher is also a good stopgap during cold winter months for women with long, thick locks that take time to dry naturally or who lack access to a bonnet dryer.

Make no mistake, this is a temporary alternative to a real shampoo. Once your natural sebum has begun to turn, a refresher may not last more than a couple of days before you are again fighting the urge to scratch in public.

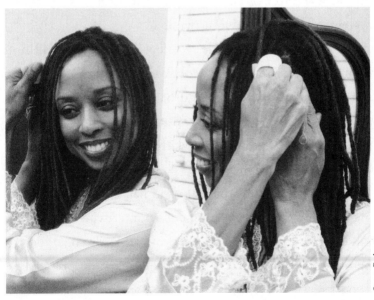

Steve Roberts

## LOCKING METHODS AND SHAMPOOING

The first problem you must make peace with is that, in the beginning, some or many of your palm-rolled coils will un-coil when you shampoo. This is a fact of locking you just have to accept and be prepared to deal with as part of the process. No use in calling up the salon/loctician and wail-ing about how "when I washed them, they all came out." So what. Coil them back up.

If you are starting your locks with two-strand twists or braids, you will have less retwisting to do, but you will still need to retwist any twists that come loose. After condition-ing, give the rest of your twists a light palm-rolling to en-courage the cylindrical intertwining.

Let's also face up to the fact that initially, you will not shampoo your hair every day or every other day. Now this is not to be confused with the urban myth that you will go several weeks or months without shampooing your hair. Does the idea of going about with a dirty head of hair and an itchy scalp appeal to you?

The idea is to keep the scalp and hair clean while allow-ing time for the hairs in each coil to intertwine enough to hold the lock together. It is that simple. Daily shampooing before this has occurred will slow or halt the process. A good rule of thumb is to shampoo your hair when it feels dirty but before it becomes just plain nasty. Five to ten days is a general estimate. Eventually, you will begin to see some coil retention after shampooing and drying. Then you can get a little froggish and jump into the shower and douse your head more often.

I wash my hair with Dr. Bronner's liquid castile soaps, which are scented with essential oils—almond, lavender, peppermint, tea tree, or eucalyptus—and an unscented baby soap. I find it interesting that the manufacturer doesn't formally recommend that this liquid soap be used as a shampoo, but they acknowledge that many people—especially curly-haired people—use it as such. I prefer Dr. Bronner's lavender liquid soap for its soothing properties and its refreshing fragrance in the hair. Dr. Bronner's peppermint liquid soap is good too—just don't get any in your eyes. The liquid soap can be diluted with water; in fact, the manufacturer suggests that you do so. Diluting the soap makes it easier to rinse from the hair, and the goals of basic lock care are to keep the locks clean and supple and to minimize residue. Castile soaps and shampoos, meaning soap products made only with olive oil, are mild and efficient cleansers.

You will discover that once you begin working with your virgin hair, you'll be able to assess the efficiency of products much more efficiently.

One of the best tips I've heard is to treat your locks as if they were an exquisite silk garment. Would you wash your fine silk garment every day? Would you wear your fine silk every day for a month without washing it? Would you throw your fine silk clothing into a hot water wash along with the sheets, towels, and your strongest detergent? Would you then put the wad of boiled silk into a hot dryer to tumble around until it was steam-baked?

**Shampoo Tools**
- Detachable showerhead
- Plastic clips
- Liquid castile soap such as Dr. Bronner's or your preferred shampoo (but avoid shampoo-conditioner combinations)

## How to Shampoo Budding or Baby Locks

First, invest in a detachable showerhead. This will allow you to rinse your scalp thoroughly by soaking it area by area with water.

After soaking first your scalp, then your hair, apply shampoo.

Spread your fingers and work the pads of your fingers into your hair until your palms and finger pads are flat against your scalp. Use the pads of your fingers to massage the shampoo onto your scalp. Don't rake the scalp with the fingernails; all this does is scratch and irritate your scalp and disturb the base of your budding locks more than necessary. (This is an extremely hair-friendly method of shampooing even if your hair is not locked.)

## How to Shampoo Mature and Long Locks

For long locks, I find it is more effective to shampoo your hair while standing in the shower unless you have someone helping you shampoo over a bathtub or large sink.

Soak your hair thoroughly with water. Bring your hair forward over each shoulder. It will be easier to handle your locks and see that you are applying shampoos and conditioners evenly and rinsing them out thoroughly.

Pour shampoo into your palms and rub your hands together to distribute it evenly between them. Work the shampoo into the scalp using the flat pads of the fingers and palms of the hands.

If you are using a liquid castile soap such as Dr. Bronner's, you can dilute the product with water, put some in a small squeeze bottle, and squirt directly onto your scalp—say, a squirt at each temple, your crown, and the nape of your neck. Then work the shampoo into the scalp using the method I've described above.

When you are satisfied that your scalp is clean, work the shampoo into the locked portion of your hair. This is when the analogy of the silk garment comes into play. Squeeze the shampoo into your locks as if you were laundering a fine knit, distributing it throughout with the palms of your hands.

When you are ready to rinse, use the detachable shower-head to soak your scalp and locks. Soak and squeeze your locks until the water runs clear. This will take several rinses and more than a few minutes, but it is an extremely important grooming habit to master if you want your locks to remain in top condition.

### ALTERNATIVE METHOD FOR LONG HAIR

You can separate your locks into four sections using wide plastic clips and then shampoo your locks section by section.

You won't have to be too concerned with the locked portion of your hair tangling unless your locks are extremely small—Sisterlocks would probably fit into this category. However, you must take care to ensure that the unlocked hair at the base of your locks is not allowed to tangle; this is to prevent the bases of the individual locks from creeping together.

The most important area to focus your shampoo and attention on is your scalp. Keep the scalp clean, and your locks will pretty much be all right. If your scalp is troubled, you're going to have unmanageable buildup in your locks. Note the expression *unmanageable buildup* because, as I've mentioned before, a small amount of residue may migrate to the core of the lock, but the goal is to minimize it so it becomes neither an aesthetic issue nor a breeding ground for odor.

## ACIDIC RINSES

Acidic rinses help close the cuticle of the hair shaft, which strengthens it and discourages product residues and soap scum. Apply the rinse immediately after shampooing. Use acidic rinses periodically but not so often that they dry out your locks. Fill a large plastic pitcher with 1 quart cool water and add 1 cup cider vinegar or the juice of one or two lemons. Saturate your locks with the rinse, let it sit for one minute, and rinse thoroughly with tepid water. Follow with your choice of conditioning treatment.

## HOT OIL TREATMENTS

For deep conditioning, nothing beats the time-tested hot oil treatment. It is the most efficient method of ensuring that your locks get what they need without fear of buildup. I fill a squeeze bottle from the beauty supply shop with olive oil from the supermarket. After shampooing, I towel-blot my locks and squeeze the oil through it, working it through with my fine silk stroke. I pop a disposable plastic shower cap over my locks and put a heating conditioning cap over it for about thirty minutes. Do some knitting, read a book, watch TV. Then I hop into the shower, lather up with Dr. Bronner's Lavender Liquid Soap—I use it undiluted after I do the hot oil treatment—and shampoo no less than twice but usually three or four times, depending on how much oil I used.

- You can give your locks a hot oil treatment every other shampoo. The only caveat is that you give your locks a couple of good lathers to remove the excess oil.
- If you absolutely must use a blow dryer on your hair, a hot oil treatment beforehand is a good hedge against drying out your locks.
- If you plan to wear a silk blouse or dress, don't give your locks a hot oil treatment on the same day; do it the day before.

## CONDITIONERS

The important quality for commercial conditioners, aside from moisturizing and protecting your locks, is that they perform this basic task with a minimum of residue. To test before you buy, discreetly rub a drop between your hands; if it disappears without much of a trace, it will generally behave that way on your locks. Conditioners designed for color-treated and extra-dry hair tend to be effective because they are moisturizers, but be sure the packaging specifies that the product doesn't leave buildup. You probably want to avoid the heavy, creamy types of "deep" conditioners because they are designed to coat the hair shaft and leave some sort of residue behind. Leave-in formulas with a watery, fluid consistency are okay because they are less likely to leave a visible residue in your locks. As long as you avoid excessive blow-drying, the main requirements for conditioning your locks are moisturizing and lubrication. Tapping into online chats and the grapevine for product recommendations can be useful.

# Three

## The Wind in Your Hair: Drying Your Locks

I've read, mostly—okay, always—in magazine features directed toward Caucasian women, countless stories illustrating a proper haircut with a freshly shampooed head of hair combed into shape, perhaps finished with a light application of mousse or styling gel. The woman will then grab her keys and run to work, see the kids off, do errands, or whatever. There is always a picture of Ms. Upwardly Mobile Thang, tendrils of comb-slicked hair framing her face, with a smattering of lip gloss, wearing a chic trench coat, hailing a cab. She'll have a smile on her face, knowing that in time, her hair will dry in the shape into which it was cut. An hour or so later, she can fluff or shake it out, freshen her lip gloss, and meet her coworkers or friends for lunch.

Years ago, I'd read this stuff, look at the pictures, and, on a bad day, feel bad that the hairdressers I knew insisted that my hair was too nappy not to be straightened (within an inch of its life) before being cut. And once it had been straightened and cut, there was no way it could be styled without being set on rollers or "bumped," which was curling the ends of my hair with a curling iron. This bumping invariably included bumping the hot iron against my forehead or temples or neck to catch the kitchen that had managed to spring through the broken, overprocessed hair on my nape. I would then carry the mark of the hair slave, the brand of the curling iron, until it healed, in time for the next touch-up. Back then, the only effect an air drying would have had on my hair was to transform it into a crackling, desiccated helmet.

I never thought I'd ever experience the sensation of sitting outside when the weather is warm, running my fingers through my hair, and allowing the sun to do its natural magic. Wearing locked hair has made a fantasy come true, with none of the downsides fantasies often have. Simply put, I can leave the house with wet hair, with a slick of lip gloss, and if the weather is warm, my hair will be dry—and presentable—in less than an hour. The only concern is that it is not dripping wet when I am out and about so I don't soak my clothes or the back of the car seat.

I live in a region with extremely hot summers, and even though we have central air conditioning at our house, my husband is addicted to the hum of electric fans, which, in fact, diffuse the cooled air efficiently. I shampoo my hair early in the day and let it air dry inside my house with the help of overhead and spot fans. When I have errands to run, I drive with the car windows open; I call this my mobile hair dryer.

When my locks were budding and in the teen stage, I would dry them after they'd been palm rolled with gel and held in place with metal clips. I found that several minutes under a hooded dryer set the gelled coils enough so I could let the locks air dry without worrying they'd unfurl. My portable hooded hair dryer has been one of my smartest hair investments. It wasn't expensive; I bought mine at a discount retailer, and they are readily available at beauty supply stores. As my locks have continued to grow, I use the bonnet dryer during cold months when air drying may not be the best option. I'm pretty conservative when it comes to heat settings and suggest you avoid overheating your own hair. Many bonnet dryers have a special heat setting for wigs—this is usually a safe bet and won't dry out my locks.

I wick as much excess moisture as possible from my locks. A super-absorbent hair towel is a handy tool that will help cut down air drying time. These towels are made of microfibers that absorb many times their weight in water. Look for them in beauty supply stores or wherever bedding and linen are sold. They are a fairly inexpensive investment, which is good, because as your locks grow longer you will need two or three to do the job. The most effective way to use them is to blot the excess moisture from your locks by squeezing a towel over a handful of locks at a time. Use the same action you would if you were squeezing water from a delicate knit or washable silk. Wringing out your locks like a pair of socks is likely to do the same thing it would do to a delicate knit: pull the meshed coils apart, causing weak spots and thinning within individual locks.

I use hair dryers only to *help* dry my locks, never to dry them completely. Whenever I did a full-bore bake under the bonnet, my locks came out dryer, harder, started lying all funny on my head—in short, all the bugaboos of my over-processed hair days came back in waves, and I'd come too far to go back to that. Because my hair was unprocessed, I could see the effects of my shortsighted laziness immediately, and my hair responded just as immediately to proper

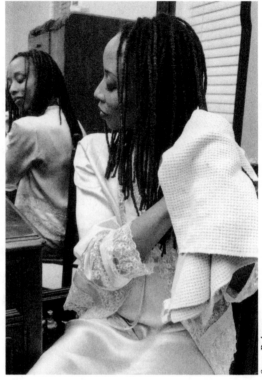

Steve Roberts

care—which just wouldn't have happened had my hair been overprocessed.

Keeping my locks supple is the best way to ensure that they remain on my head. I've seen hard broom-dry dreads and have sworn that that wasn't to be the fate of mine.

I use a blow-dryer only to hasten or finish drying my hair, not for the whole job, as blow-drying can really dry out your locks in no time. If you absolutely must blow-dry (let's say it's 30 degrees outside and you have to be at work in a half-hour), then follow these simple rules to do it safely. First, blot as much moisture from your locks as possible, then use the blow-dryer on a low setting, no higher than medium. A diffuser is safer but it does slow down the process, and it tends to lull me into a false sense of security where I might use the blow-dryer longer than is necessary. Keep the dryer moving constantly or you'll scorch your locks. Concentrate on the hair closest to your scalp because the ends of your locks will dry fastest—and remember that the ends of your locks are the part that must be protected at all costs.

When the weather is warm, you can sit outside with your back to the sun and let solar heat do the work for you. If you have a hankering to lighten your hair, here's the perfect opportunity to apply a lightening rinse and let nature take its course. Remember to compensate for the slightly drying effects of lighteners and apply some oil moisturizer while the hair is still damp. If you need it, add a bit more after your locks are dry.

# Four

## Tending Your Garden: Locked Hair Care

Locks are probably the simplest (not to be confused with quickest and easiest) way to groom hair you'll ever experience. Keep the scalp clean, encourage the coils to twine into locks, keep them from creeping (see page 71), and keep them supple. That's it.

Make your hair routine simple, and it will be easy to follow. A relaxing and beneficial hair routine can include a daily (or nightly) five-minute scalp massage with the pads of your fingers, followed by an application of a light oil treatment for your locks once or twice a week.

## Basic Gear for Locked Hair

- **Holding agent or alcohol-free gel.** Look for products marketed for locks or braids.
- **Metal hair clips,** to hold freshly palm-rolled locks in place while drying.
- **Metal-free elastic bands,** to separate and hold the locks you're not working on out of the way during grooming sessions.
- A **thimble,** to measure oil smoothed through your locks.
- **Your choice of moisturizing oils or hair moisturizer.** The best oils for your scalp and locks are of organic and botanic origin. Use any oil you would use to moisturize your skin. Mineral oil and petroleum-based oils should be avoided as they irritate the scalp, cause flaking, and promote buildup. I've listed some of the products I use in the Resources section of this book.
- A **small apothecary of essential oils** for your scalp. I have these basics on hand; they are inexpensive and commonly available. Choose the small, dark bottles usually sold at health or natural foods stores, because

essential oils have a short shelf life and should probably be replaced regularly. *Do a 24-hour skin test on the
inside of your wrist to test for skin sensitivity. People with
epilepsy and pregnant women should consult a doctor before using essential oils.*

- *Rosemary*—astringent, retards flaking, stimulates
  scalp and follicles, promotes sheen in dark hair.
- *Tea tree*—antiseptic, antifungal.
- *Lavender*—soothing, prevents blistering and scar-
  ring, promotes healing of skin and scalp irritation,
  relieves itching.
- *Sage*—antiseptic, retards flaking, good for dark
  hair. Should not be used by pregnant women.

- **Skin antiseptics** such as witch hazel, tea tree oil, or Sea
  Breeze.
- **Cheesecloth or gauze pads** for refreshing or cleaning
  the scalp with antiseptics.
- A **collection of silk, satin, or acetate scarves** to protect
  your hair while you sleep.
- **Plastic shower caps.** Yeah, freedom hair can stand up
  to moisture, but you don't want to saturate your locks
  in the shower every day unless you are in a climate
  that promotes quick and thorough drying. Shower

caps are also necessary for hot oil treatments. Buy them in economical bulk at beauty supply stores.

- A **heated conditioning cap.** Indispensable for hot oil treatments. No more wet towels. Available at beauty supply stores.

- A **bonnet-style hair dryer.** Optional but a boon to have, a bonnet dryer can be a lifesaver when the weather is cold, your locks are too damp to stand the chill, and your time is short. The dryer can also be used to set a fresh palm-rolling and clip session. Just remember that it is intended as a *finishing* tool and not to bake your locks from drippy wet to crispy dry.

- A **collection of hair accessories.** Hair sticks, clips, metal-free elastics. Pretty scarves to tie up your hair. Chic hats and soft wool caps to protect your locks from cold winters and hot sun.

## GROOMING

This is a good time for a talk about Nappy Hair Phobia. Some people prefer looking new and tight around the roots, with the unlocked hair in a shiny, tight, oiled, gelled coil, scalp visible at the partings. Others prefer not to see their scalp shining through the partings and enjoy a sort of

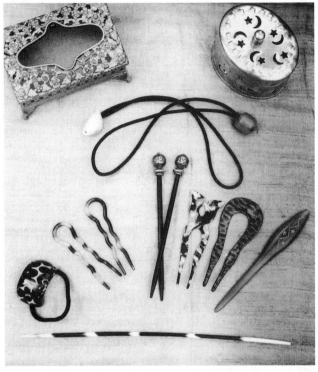

Steve Roberts

controlled nappy coiliness with well-cared-for locks. What-ever floats your boat.

My feeling has always been that locks are the supreme triumph of form following function—that is to say, locked hair is the manifestation of intertwined coils, the fruit of the nappy root. Therefore, there's no sense in constant twisting every time a nap pops up. If you ain't down with the aes-thetic, then you should probably put off the notion of lock-ing your hair until you are.

That being said, the tangible danger of twisting every time your roots look the least bit real is that you will weaken and thin the base of your locks and cause them to break off. The thinning of the lock shaft will occur at the base or appear further down the shaft as a weak spot.

## The Importance of Popping Your Locks

Locked hair is like a garden; if you don't weed it regularly, everything grows between the rows and you won't be able to tell where the weeds end and the garden begins. All you'll know is that it's a mess and it's growing on your head. Keeping your locks separated is referred to as *popping*. The locks are simply separated at each shampooing or when the hair has been dampened. The locks are pulled apart from each other at the base so separate locks will not grow together (unless you *want* them to marry—see "Locking 911"). The term *popping* comes from the sound the hair makes when you pull the locks apart. Popping often sounds like you're ripping your hair out, but you won't unless you've neglected your locks for so long that you need scissors to cut apart married locks.

**Creeping** happens when locks are not routinely separated after shampooing; visualize weeds in a garden. The individual separation at the base of each lock is gone, and locks begin to grow together or marry at the base. It's never too late to correct creeping, unless the creeping has begun to mat. Give your locks a shampoo and conditioning oil treatment. Grab the locking gel/aloe vera/whatever you like, some hair clips, sit yourself down, and start popping and rolling those locks. Keep the unlocked hair damp until you've popped and separated your entire head. Be gentle but firm.

**Matting** is the terminal outcome of creeping, where the separation is nonexistent and the unlocked hair is hopelessly meshed. Visualize a short, matted afro with locks floating on top. You will need a loctician's help or several hours with a diligent friend whose commitment to locks is stronger than yours. You may want to reexamine your professed desire for locked hair. You must consider the possibility that you may have to grow another set of locks.

### The Gospel of Lock Grooming

- **Always** dampen locks before rolling, popping, or twisting.
- **Never** rub your hands back and forth; always roll the hair in one continuous motion between your palms.
- **Never sleep on wet or damp locks.** Sleeping on wet locks can cause them to lose their cylindrical shape and flatten, like linguine. Binding damp or wet locks under tight scarves or hats will also flatten them. Once a lock

flattens (also referred to as *flapping*), there isn't a whole lot you can do to restore it to a completely cylindrical shape; however, you can prevent future flapping by being sure to palm-roll your locks regularly.

- **Palm-roll your hair in one direction.** Decide whether you want to twist toward your face or away from your face and stick to it. Here's a way to keep the direction of your roll consistent:

  Envision that your hair is parted from the middle, from your hairline to the nape of your neck. Twist all the locks on one side toward or away from your face. Do the same with the other side.

  Decide how you want the locks that frame your face to fall, but know that you pretty much need to set a pattern and stick to it. The hair at your hairline is delicate, and twisting it in different directions at every grooming session will snap it off.

## GROOMING TIMETABLE

Once your locks are sufficiently established, your general grooming schedule should go something like this:

**After each shampoo,** separate and pop your locks and simply *turn* them in the direction they should lie.

**Every two or three weeks,** separate, pop, and palm-twist new growth. You don't have to make tight rolls; an encouraging pass between your palms will help keep things in line between more thorough grooming sessions.

**Every six weeks,** separate, pop, and palm-twist using a holding gel and clips to hold the palm-rolled new growth until dry. Think of it as a touch-up, except that this touch-up isn't going to burn your scalp and you get to keep the hair you grew in the six weeks since the last touch-up.

As you get to know your own hair, you can adjust this timeline to suit your own needs.

## MASSAGE

A five-minute scalp massage every day will do wonders for the circulation in the scalp and encourage maximum hair growth. Five minutes is manageable for virtually everyone, and for coily hair, massage is far superior to daily brushing with a hundred strokes. In fact, as discussed at length in my book *Good Hair: For Colored Girls Who've Considered Weaves When the Chemicals Became Too Ruff,* brushing techniques intended for naturally straight hair can encourage coily hair strands to snap.

To massage your scalp, you must position your hands and fingers so that the *pads* of the fingers, not the *nails,* make contact with your scalp.

Spread your fingers as shown in the photograph. Work the fingers into the hair so that the pads of the fingers lie on the scalp. Use the pads of the fingers to make circular motions on the skin of the scalp, not the hair itself. The pads of the fingers should make contact with the scalp as if you were bald. You can pinch and lift the skin and gently move the scalp back and forth to loosen it.

When the circulation is stimulated, the nutrients that nourish the roots of the hair are absorbed more efficiently. Think of massage as sowing a fertile scalp that will yield the healthiest locks possible.

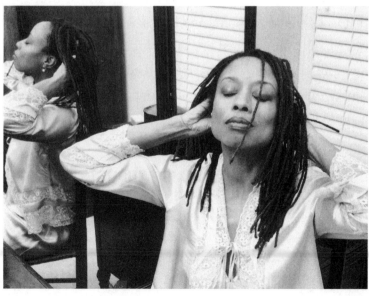

Steve Roberts

## LIGHT OIL TREATMENTS: KEEPING LOCKED HAIR SUPPLE

Once or twice a week, following your daily five-minute scalp massage, indulge in a light oil treatment to keep locks supple.

Fill your thimble with oil, pour the oil into your palms, and rub your hands together to coat them evenly. Take a small section of locks—maybe ten at a time, depending on their thickness. Stroke your oiled palms gently but firmly down the length of the section of locks. Remember, less is more, and it is better to use oil by the thimbleful and be stingy with it than to saturate the locks with so much oil that it stains your clothing and linens. It may be a good rule not to use your best bed linens the night after any oil treatment, in case your locks have absorbed a lot of oil, the excess of which will end up staining your pillowcase and being ground into your facial skin.

## COMMERCIAL CONDITIONING PRODUCTS

A wide variety of commercial products is designed for locks, braids, and twists. For example, you can use organic botanic oils for deep conditioning and oil moisturizing. You can try oil moisturizing hair lotions to keep your locks

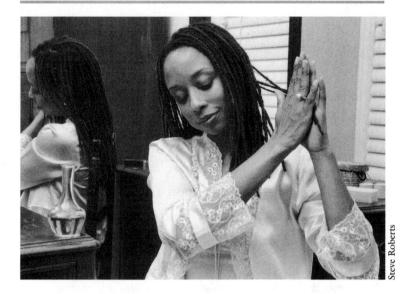

Steve Roberts

supple and botanical treatments for itchy and dry scalp. My recommendation is to key the product(s) you like into your hair care system. Streamline your routine and spend your money on a favorite hair oil rather than trying and rejecting bottles of the latest hair cure-all. Read labels and be selective. My basic recommendation is to avoid products containing beeswax, mineral oil, and petrolatum.

## NIGHTTIME LOCK CARE

Once upon a time, I believed that once my hair was locked, I could toss gently while in deep slumber, hair tumbled across the pillow, just like the white girls I saw in the movies. No more nights of reaching up to pat my head in my sleep to ensure that my head rag, that literal bondage of womanly negritude, was still in place. I discovered that my notion of bondage was poppycock and that scarf-free could very well mean being lock-free.

As my buds began to mesh into young locks, I wanted to keep them neat, so I tied them up at night. The first year and a half of locking my hair, I wanted to keep the fuzz factor down and was diligent about keeping my locks tied up at night. Then I became lazy about covering my hair. I rationalized my laziness: *Seven nights a week underneath a scarf was stifling my scalp, it was a bit flaky, it needed airing.* It was also a bit of throwing my fist into the air to protest against what I perceived as hair bondage; what was I locking my hair for if not to escape wearing a rag on my head to bed? It was during this period of sleeping scarf-free that I noticed my locks seemed dry only a few days after shampooing and a hot oil treatment. An informal poll of locked friends and acquaintances gave me the answer I wasn't especially keen on hearing, but the feel of rough, dry locks against my skin spoke much louder. They told me that if I didn't get with the program and cover my hair at night that my husband would not appreciate touching locks that felt like stiff wool.

As far as the flakiness was concerned, I discovered that the scarves were not the culprit. I simply began to shampoo and rinse more carefully, massaged and moisturized my scalp, and changed my scarves when they stopped smelling fresh. Bonus: Covering your locks at night also helps minimize lint deposits.

When I sleep, I take care that my hair is arranged in such a way that when I tie my scarf around it, it hangs down my back.

So the moral of this story is to put together a wardrobe of scarves so you can rotate your head rags. After all, would you wear the same clothes day after day? It's perfectly acceptable to slip your scarf under your pillow before you make your love connection. Later, when you're ready to go to sleep, under the cover of darkness, you slip it back on your head and everybody's happy. Put your locks to bed at night so you'll have lush and supple locks to swing over your shoulder tomorrow.

## MAXIMUM GROWTH

Once your locks have matured—say, about a year after you've begun locking—the best is yet to come. It is now time to get a pretty journal and a soft or cloth tape measure.

Stand up and make sure your hair is pulled back from your hairline and hanging back or over your shoulders if it is long. The most accurate way to measure your hair is from your hairline at the forehead in the center. Put the end of the tape in the middle of your forehead at your hairline. If your hair is long, let the tape fall down the middle of your back to where your hair ends. If your hair is layered, measure to the end of the longest locks.

If your hair is long and you cannot turn your head around far enough behind you to read the measurement from the mirror, hold the tape a couple of inches above where the tape measure ends, making sure your locks are straight against the tape. Holding the ends of your locks and the tape measure, pull both around so you can see them.

Try to measure your hair at regular intervals; once a month is a good yardstick. Keep a record of your measurements in your journal along with information like trims and any observations about your hair care routine or diet.

## MAINTAINING THE LENGTH OF YOUR LOCKS

It is possible to maintain your locks successfully for years with timely hot oil treatments (see page 57 in "How Do

You Wash Them?," for instructions), scalp massage, seasonal protection from the elements, and a reasonably healthy lifestyle. It simply takes the systematic commitment to do what is necessary to achieve the results you desire—beautiful locked hair.

- **Inspect your locks regularly for weak or thinning spots.** Ideally, you want to nip this in the bud, literally. That is, if you spot a thinning section near the tip of the lock, you can snip it off. Better to snip $\frac{1}{16}$ or $\frac{1}{2}$ inch of lock than to have a larger length break off. If the weak spot is farther up the lock, you can shore it up with a sew-and-wrap method and some kinky human hair extension. See "Locking 911" for suggestions on how to do this.

- **Massage your scalp every day for at least five minutes, ideally ten.** Massage stimulates circulation, which delivers nutrients to your scalp. As you massage, so shall you reap.

- **Eat a well-balanced diet** so the nutrients you ingest will be fed into your bloodstream.

- **Get trims only when you need them and only to remove damaged ends of your locks.** Don't follow the old rule about mandatory trims every six weeks; instead, use that guideline to inspect your locks for damage, lint, etc., and take care of these problems on a lock-by-lock basis. Free your mind!

- **Treat your locks like fine silk.** Resist the temptation to take shortcuts like lengthy hot blow-drying sessions because you didn't plan your time wisely.

## Five

### Locking 911

Try to remember, above all, that the great advantages of wearing locked hair are that you can head off a lot of problems before they are irreversible and that you can repair individual locks in a way that is impossible to do with unlocked hair. Consider this: If unlocked hair is plagued with split ends, the only alternative is to stave off a trim with cosmetic conditioning treatments or cut the hair. A damaged lock can be repaired, reattached, or intertwined with a stronger lock. Note that this can be done using one's own lock.

Finally, consider that even in the worst-case scenario, your hair will grow back and that you can lock your hair again with confidence, knowing that in time you will have tangible results flowing down your shoulders, if that is what you desire. For many of us, this is a priceless delight and a comfort that was unattainable when our hair was processed.

Use this chapter as a troubleshooting reference for locks, a quick guide to common locked-hair emergencies, with panic-free solutions you can manage.

## DANDRUFF

Every thing that flakes is not dandruff. If you think you have dandruff, examine your scalp. Mild but annoying flaking could be the residue from styling products like gels or sprays. It can even be residue from conditioners that weren't rinsed out properly. Petroleum- or mineral-based hair lubricants can also cause the scalp to flake because they tend to be irritating. For that reason, I've found that vegetable- and plant-based oils are best for hair and scalp care. Try clarifying shampoos (shampoos designed to remove buildup) or switching to products other than the ones you've been using before checking out dandruff shampoos.

Severe, heavy flaking and itching, accompanied by a reddened scalp and/or pus, requires a dermatologist's care.

### Dandruff Remedies

- **Tea tree oil** added to a mild castile shampoo or soap, such as Dr. Bronner's liquid castile soaps.
- **Commercially prepared dandruff shampoos.** Avoid coal tar dandruff shampoos and dandruff relief products, however, because coal tar is a suspected carcinogen.
- **Rosemary, lavender, avocado, sage, jojoba, calendula, or birch essential oils.** Apply undiluted to itchy and flaky spots as long as the skin isn't broken. Add a few drops to carrier oils (these are base oils such as almond, grapeseed, or olive to which you add therapeutic essential oils). You can also try botanical commercial oils and scalp treatments marketed to relieve itchy, flaky scalps. Read those labels; remember to avoid mineral oil, because that will worsen the problem.

## BUILDUP

If you cut a lock and examine the cross section, you will probably see a whitish deposit at the core. This comes from minute quantities of lint and product buildup. Reasonably well maintained locks should have less of this material at the core.

If you've gone for quick cosmetic crutches like beeswax or have been indiscriminately using products containing petrolatum in an effort to make your locks shine, the buildup in the deep core will be heavy and will permeate each lock. Heavy core buildup will dry and stiffen locked hair.

When your locks look grayish and dusty, surface buildup is usually the culprit. Take a smell check to make sure mildew isn't the culprit. Surface buildup results from an accumulation of several factors: dirt and scalp effluvia, beeswax and petroleum products, lazy shampoo and rinsing techniques, and conditioners that are intended for unlocked hair and leave a heavy film.

- **Prevention**—When it comes to shampooing, err on the side of cleanliness. If your scalp is dirty enough to require shampooing twice in one week, then shampoo twice a week, although you can probably get away with a scalp refresher or a rinse. Keep the dirt on your scalp to a minimum.
- **Product buildup removal**—Wash your hair with a clarifying shampoo. Product descriptions vary from com-

pany to company; look for keywords such as "removes buildup."

- **Heavy buildup removal** such as that caused by beeswax and petrolatum products—Try using a clarifying shampoo followed by an acidic rinse. See chapter 3 for instructions on acidic rinses. Squeeze the acidic solution through your locks for ten minutes and rinse with the hottest water you can stand without burning your scalp. Your locks will be parched after this, so recondition them with a thirty- to sixty-minute deep-conditioning hot oil treatment.

## WEAKENED LOCKS

Weak spots along the shaft of a lock are usually due to over-twisting (twisting your locks much more frequently than necessary) or twisting the locks when dry. Both of these actions stretch and break the coiled strands that are spun into each lock. The broken coils intertwine with the rest of the lock but the weak spot remains like a gap in the weave of fabric. Starting locks that are micro-thin also puts them at risk for breakage.

- **Sit on your hands and stop twisting for a few weeks** so the new growth can thicken and strengthen.

- **Examine your locks regularly** and remember the golden rule: Spindly locks are delicate locks, so examination is twice as important. A lock that thins drastically in spots along the shaft is a lock with a high probability of breakage.

- **Consider shotgunning (or marrying) thin locks.** The idea is to splice the weak lock to a stronger lock or splice two weak locks together for strength. Yeah, instead of three locks you'll have two, but you were gonna lose a lock with nothing to show for it anyway. Why not reincarnate it and strengthen your locks to boot?

  Take the thin lock and choose a lock next to it; it can be the same size or larger. First, you must splice together the roots of the two locks so they will grow from the same base. To do this, open a hole in the loose hair at the base of one lock and thread the entire length of the other lock through the hole. Then intertwine the free lengths of the two locks so they mesh together into a single lock. To do this, twist the locks into a single two-lock twist. Take care to maintain married locks so they don't separate or fork at the ends.

- **Shore up weak sections of individual locks** with strands of natural or kinky-textured extension hair. To do this, thread several strands of extension hair through a needle (you can use a hair-weaving needle from a beauty supply store or find a suitable sewing needle). Treat the extension hair like thread. Alternately stitch and wrap the extension hair around the weak or thinned area to reinforce it. When you've reinforced the lock to your liking, trim the ends of any extension hairs that protrude from the lock. The goal is to darn the lock using the extension hair, which ideally will blend in with the texture of your lock as it ages.

- **Forked locks** (locks with one base but two ends) can be repaired by joining the ends with extension hair.

## Lock Replacement

- **Save detached locks if at all possible.** Even if locks are lost due to hair pulling or other mayhem, it is often possible to recover them when the dust settles.

- **Reattach locks that are broken at the root** by braiding the lock into the unlocked base hair. You can wait until your base hair is long enough to braid and do it yourself or have a braider do it for you.

- **Bond locks with hair bond**—yes, the product they use for bond weaves and extensions. Bonding is a better alternative for locks that break farther down the shaft.

If you choose this method for locks that broke closer to the root, keep in mind that the point where the lock is rejoined may feel a bit hard due to the bonding agent and will remain so until your lock grows long enough to be cut. Locticians and cosmetologists that specialize in hair extension can perform this service for you.

## LINT

Lint is a benign nuisance that can be minimized by daily inspection and maintenance of your locks.

- Pick out **isolated cases of embedded lint** with a pair of pointed tweezers.
- Deal with **hopelessly embedded isolated spots of lint** by altering the color of the lint—*the lint itself and not the lock*—with a black or brown Sanford Sharpie Permanent Marker.
- Cosmetically remedy a **proliferation of lint** throughout your locks by coloring or dying your hair. Be aware that frequent lock coloring has built-in hazards, discussed in detail in the chapter on coloring.

## MILDEW

Sleeping on damp locks and developing residue buildup that retains moisture will encourage your locks to sour and mildew.

- **Saturate your locks** (not your scalp) with an alcohol-based antiseptic like Sea Breeze. You can also add several drops of tea tree oil to 4 cups of warm water and saturate your locks with the solution. Squeeze the antiseptic or solution through your locks as if you were laundering a fine silk or knit garment. Allow it to remain in the locks for five minutes and then shampoo with a clarifying shampoo. Remember that clarifying shampoo formulas are designed to remove buildup. Rinse until the water runs clear.

- **Shampoo with tea tree–enhanced cleansers** such as Dr. Bronner's liquid tea tree soap.

# Six

## Coloring

I have always admired the way women who wore locks were rather fearless and creative with the color of their hair. In addition to coal-black and chocolate locks I love seeing just about every imaginable shade in nature and then some. Silvery white, auburns, true reds, cherry reds, heathery grays, caramel blondes, golden browns highlighted with golden streaks, burgundy, blue highlights—there's something about locks that releases the adventuress in every woman.

Adventures in coloring locked hair are best left to professional colorists—but be aware that there are risks even with professionals. I have heard and seen the results of horror stories of women who have had to cut their locks back to bud stage because the colorist overprocessed their locks and they literally broke off. The problem is that often, the coloring solution penetrates the core of the locks and cannot completely be rinsed out. The chemicals remain embedded in the locks, where they weaken and dry out the shaft. Blonde shades are especially tricky; lightening the hair takes longer to process, so the chemicals are especially likely to penetrate the locks.

If you are considering light brown or blonde shades, do a lot of legwork and check up on the colorist's success rate with locked hair before you sit in the chair.

Have your colorist use a semipermanent hair coloring, one that is designed to shampoo out gradually. Semipermanent coloring has a shorter processing time, so the coloring agent is less likely to penetrate your locks to the point where it is impossible to completely remove it.

## LESS INVASIVE COLORING METHODS FOR LOCKED HAIR

Try simply *enhancing* your hair color. Color glazes are semipermanent coloring agents; one well-known brand is

Jazzing by Clairol. Glazes don't contain ammonia or peroxide, so the damage quotient is lessened. These clear color glazes or glosses are designed to deposit a shiny transparent color that will shampoo out gradually; however, on locked hair, you won't get a shine. Deeper shades of glaze can enrich your color, but you must rinse very thoroughly. Don't expect to lighten your natural hair color with these products. Your best bet is to have a colorist apply color glaze.

Enhancing your hair color with home brews such as those described here isn't as dramatic as commercial hair coloring, but it isn't as potentially damaging either. Still, you must compensate for the drying effects of the rinses with regular hot oil treatments. With the exception of the Chamomile-Lemon Sun Rinse, the rinses can be used when you feel your color needs a lift. The Sun Rinse is a mild bleaching agent, so use it once during the summer, and if it brightens your hair, you can try it again the next summer.

## Darkening Rinses

Apply the rinse after shampooing, let it sit for five minutes, then rinse out. Finish with a conditioning oil and air dry if possible.

### COFFEE RINSE

2 cups inky strong coffee (cooled)

Juice of 2 lemons

Combine.

### SAGE AND TEA RINSE

$\frac{1}{2}$ cup fresh sage leaves

$\frac{1}{2}$ cup of any whole-leaf dark tea

Bring 3 cups of water to a boil, remove from heat, and pour over the sage and tea leaves. Let it steep for 1 hour or until completely cool. Strain the mixture before rinsing your locks.

## Lightening Rinses

### CHAMOMILE RINSE

1 cup chamomile tea (you can buy this in bulk at health stores)

Bring 3 cups of water to a boil, remove from heat, and steep tea for 1 hour or until cool. Strain the mixture before rinsing your locks.

## CHAMOMILE-LEMON SUN RINSE

Try this on a hot, sunny day.

Chamomile tea rinse, cooled

Juice of 4 lemons

Shampoo your hair and sit outside in the sun for the better part of an hour. Keep in mind that this acidic rinse works with the sun as an organic bleaching/lightening agent. Be careful to rinse your locks thoroughly and give your hair a hot oil treatment afterward.

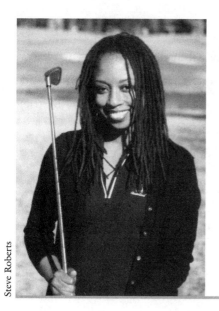

## Seven

### Working Up a Sweat

I lucked out in the genetic lottery, have never had a weight problem, and have coasted through with no regular exercise for most of my life. Folks in Memphis would look at me and ask, "How do you hold yourself in like that?" I laughed and took that to be some sort of cornpone way of asking what I did to stay in shape. I'd grin and stand just a little taller and straighter, trying to represent fitness. But when I was home alone naked in front of the bathroom mirror I realized that sooner or later, folks were gonna peep my trump card. Heck, they probably already had. Truth was, I *was* holding myself in, had been for years, but I had reached a certain age and I knew—as perpetrators who live by their wits and nothing else do—that my gig was up.

Like many sistas with intentions about exercising, I got to stuttering and mumbling when it came time to commit myself to doing something about it. Give me a reason to procrastinate and I'll take it. Most women use their hair as an excuse not to exercise: can't sweat out the perm, don't want to put their head on the floor—the litany is part of the African American woman's lexicon. In my case, my hair was both my excuse and my savior. When I decided to lock my hair, procrastination about exercise paled in light of becoming the personification of ugly-lock mythology. I could wax righteous here, blow some smoke about how people think women with locks are lesbian, depressed, unclean, or not feminine, and I felt duty bound to set a good example. I could rant about not wanting to give the Nap Patrol yet another reason to justify their crusade against hair diversity. But I'm going to keep it real; it was my own vanity that pulled me through. I didn't want to rock locked hair and not be at least halfway cute.

I knew enough to understand I couldn't achieve balance in my body if my head was off balance, trying to avoid any activity that would ruin my hairstyle. There really isn't any physical exertion that you can undertake, including golf and yoga, that will leave your hair alone. If it's hot, you're probably going to perspire. If it's cold, you're going to need to conserve body heat by covering your head. Tee off on the golf course and you'll probably need to shield your eyes from the sun with a visor, which must be worn . . . on your head. Some women flirt with the idea of practicing yoga because they have the idea that yoga is being stretched out on a mat without breaking a sweat or messing up your hair. Not if you're serious about reaping the benefits, it isn't. And I was serious about the benefits of yoga, which I

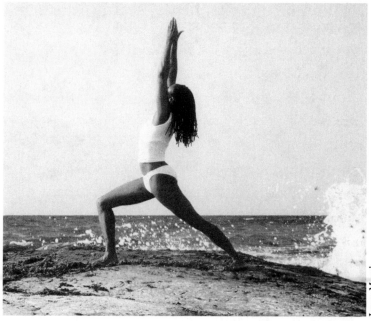

Laura Mucel

began practicing when I started locking my hair and continue to enjoy to this day.

Locked hair is made for the beach. I thought sand would stick in my locks—it didn't. The only thing I had to remember to bring on the beach with me was sunblock, a hat for shade, and a book to read. When my locks were short,

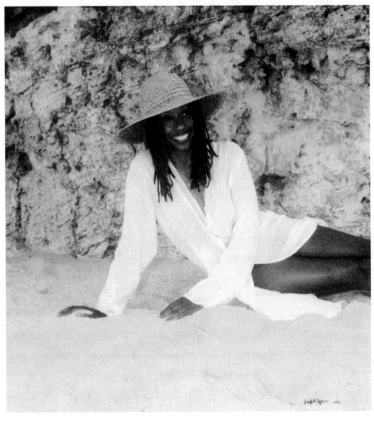

Laura Mucel

I'd swim and shake the water out of my locks. As they grew longer, I'd be sure to bring an elastic band to put them up into a sprout on the crown of my head. The next summer the sprout had lengthened into a cascade. I liked looking at snapshots of me vacationing with my family on the beach and seeing how my locks had changed length from summer to summer. I liked how I wasn't the least bit concerned about how my hair looked after I came out of the ocean, because it always looked just fine.

## SURF AND SUN CARE

While enjoying swims in the ocean or pool, periodically rinse your locks with a freshwater shower. It's a good idea to carry an extra bottle of water with you so you can douse your locks if a freshwater shower isn't available. Rinse salt or chlorinated pool water out of your hair before you settle down in the sun with a beach novel; the combination of sun and salt or chlorinated water will dry out your locks. Chlorinated water tends to discolor them as well. Always give your locks a shampoo and thorough rinse after swimming, and if you don't have time for a deep hot-oil treatment, take care to remoisturize your locks with an oil moisturizer or hair lotion afterward.

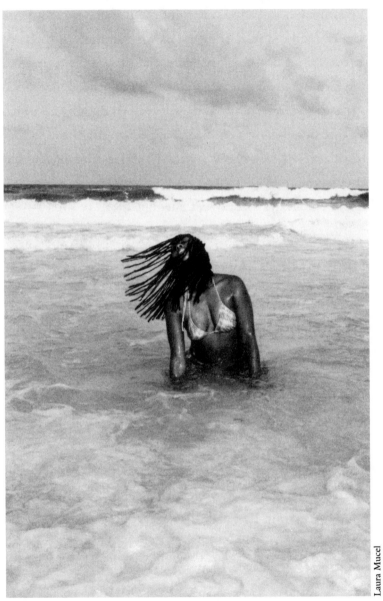

Laura Mucel

I learned to put my locks up off my neck when it was hot and to be grateful when they grew long enough to frame my face and keep my ears and neck warm when I walked through icy streets. I pop a cloche of soft mohair wool on my head, and when I get indoors I pull it off and run my fingers through my locks, give them a shake, just to fluff some air through them. I can sit down or go about my business like regular folk instead of making a panicked dash for the sanctuary of the ladies' room to make sure the life hadn't been smothered out of my do, mashed beyond repair.

Even under conditions like an advanced vinyasa class, sprawled face down into a submissive Child's Pose, dripping with sweat, my locks don't let me down because the coiliness that results from exertion integrates itself into the hairstyle at best or exaggerates the springiness at worst. A win-win hair situation if ever I saw one. The only drawback I've experienced is my locks feeling a little heavy when I worked up a good sweat on a humid day, but that is a small and temporary discomfort compared to my enjoyment from wearing them. Think of the psychological liberation that results from knowing you can enjoy physical exertion without self-consciousness about your appearance.

## PONYTAILS: WEATHERPROOF HAIR SAVIOR OR HAIRLINE BUSTER?

When I began locking my hair, I looked forward to the day when I'd be able to throw it back into a ponytail that brushed my waist and keep on sweating. The longer my locks grew, the more I realized this to be a half-baked fantasy at best. In reality, that kind of management would cost me some locks.

The placement of a *classic* ponytail puts the entire weight of your hair near the occipital bone of the cranium. This means that your hair must be firmly anchored in suspension; picture a handle with one end anchored to the back of your head. Two forces work against your hairline and temples: the tension created from the sheer weight of your hair aided by the natural law of gravity and the tension and traction created by the elastic band or fastener that contains the hair at the gathering point. This is a revelation that has caused me to be ridiculed by women who have been hair challenged as a result of nappy-hair phobia (too many touch-ups), budget braid jobs ("If I don't make it tight it won't last as long"), or habitually throwing their hands up in defeat ("I just pull it up and *pin* on a ponytail").

It doesn't matter if the ponytail is small and dinky or long and bountiful; the combination of tension and traction will result in traction alopecia marked by a gradually receding hairline. Either way, something's got to give, and it's always going to be your hairline. Always.

The safest way to wear a *classic* ponytail is not often. A better way to wear a ponytail is to place the band at the nape of the neck with slackness in the crown of the hair to avoid pulling. Another method is to gather the hair at the crown of the head—again, with great care not to pull the hair so sleekly and tightly against the skull that you get a nonsurgical facelift—and anchor it with a fastener. This method lessens direct tension at the hairline, and the head, as opposed to the hair itself, supports the weight of the ponytail.

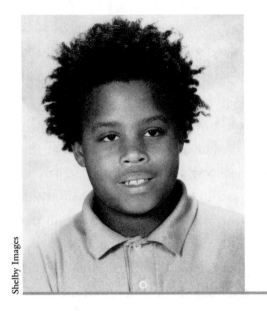

# Eight

## Manchild in the Dirty South

When my son Roland was nine years old, he wanted to begin locking his hair. I resisted the notion for a long time. My position was that the boy stayed nasty. Why walk past a puddle when he could stomp through it? What were dead leaves and grass on the ground for if he wasn't supposed to roll around in them? In the summertime, my husband, known as the Enabler, would let Roland and his buddies— the Brothers in Grime—turn the hose on in the backyard, wet down the dirt around the oak tree, and host a mud free-for-all. Water? The boy loved water. He'd spend forty minutes in the tub every night, melting and smearing bars of soap on the tiles, telling himself stories, holding his breath under water, singing, whistling, soaking towels, drowning army men, leaving a brown ring around the tub—and sure as you're reading this, emerge just as dirty as when he went in. He could wash his face and still have morning crust in his eyes, brush his teeth twice a day— that's a lot for a kid—and they'd still be as yellow as butter. There was no way he was gonna rock any locks as long as *I* had to keep them clean and twist them up.

"Mom, when do you think I could grow some locks?"

"When you can stay just a little bit cleaner . . . like when you're in high school."

In the interest of setting the record straight, the previous passage is my recollection of Roland Back When He Was a Kid. This is not Roland Today.

I had a laundry list of reasons to be against greenlighting my child's hair locking. Yes, *I* was old enough to sign up, but locking is a commitment *he*'s not old enough to make; he needs to be sure; I'm the one who'll have to keep his hair clean and groom his locks; I don't have the time. . . .

But the one reason I conveniently omitted was the projection of my own shameful cowardice—the fear that my son would be sent home with a note from the principal of his school demanding that he comb his hair, visions of him being chased home by hordes of brainwashed little handkerchief heads hounding him into his brick sanctuary like Frankenstein's monster all because he dared to be nappy. Persecuted just because he was a race man.

You're probably figuring that with my family hair history—a high intolerance for naps that has been well documented in my previous books—I would have developed a thicker skin by now. Even when Roland was as young as five and missed a couple of haircuts, my Memphis aunts would eyeball his head and mention that his cousin J.J. was getting a haircut and wouldn't Roland like to go along? Nah, said his father. His hair is okay. Boys here in Memphis don't wear their hair like that, said my aunts. So when Roland's hair began to bud they fell silent because they are gracious ladies and stand by the adage that if you have nothing nice to say, you should hold your tongue.

Roland has never really been down with haircuts. I noticed this way back, when he finally grew enough hair to justify having it cut. He didn't mind hanging out with his dad at the barbershop, but the haircut itself wasn't an experience he looked forward to. He was an extremely tenderheaded kid with an abundantly thick head of hair, so he didn't like a lot of prodding and poking. Left to his own devices, my son Roland would definitely be a free-style, organic kind of locked brotha—a Bob Marley look if you will—but until he established a baseline of cleanliness, he was going to be a free-style, manicured kind of locked young man until his mother declared otherwise.

I didn't want to commit to his grooming sessions, so his father, my husband, stepped up to the plate. He had locked his hair back in the day for a year, while in corporate America—but that's another story another time—and thought it would be a bonding experience for the both of them. He'd show him what to do, man to man.

Well, the range of Derek's skills were popping the locks and twisting them between two fingers. Soon the grooming sessions were fewer and fewer. After a while, it consisted of Daddy helping Roland shampoo his hair and Roland shaking it dry, letting the weight of the water and the natural law of centrifugal force encourage free-form lock formation. Freshly shaken and with a dose of oil moisturizer, they were passing for teen-stage locks.

When I finally got off my behind and got up in the boy's locks, it was a Code Red—a textbook case of creeping locks, practically before my eyes. They were clean, but they were a mess. He was just washing and going and it was all my fault, I had just been letting this go on, acting like we lived in New York or Amsterdam. Where was my pride, my dignity? How could I allow this to happen?

I popped and cut and popped until I gave up and trimmed the boy's hair down—way down. His father was incensed. "The boy's been growing his hair for a year!" he said. "His locks were a mess," I said. "They are not meant to look like yours," he said, "He's a boy!" He had a point. I had been focused on my rep. Roland only wanted to enjoy his hair and keep skateboarding, building forts with his buddies, and playing NBA Street on Playstation. He told me that some kids called him worm hair and said his hair looked bad but those kids thought it looked bad even when his locks were tight and looked good. He said he knew that those kids were jerks who hated nappy hair. Most people he knew thought his locks were cool and he felt good about his hair. After I scissored it down, he looked sad and said that he missed his "wild hair." I'd fallen down on the watch and let his locks creep, but the real issue was how I projected my own fears onto my son.

The lovely daughter of one of our neighbors, Lauren Fitzgerald, began to twist Roland's locks whenever she came to babysit him. She admires locks and enjoyed helping cultivate them. Soon Roland's rugged head of locks, suitable to his persona as a rugged young man, came back. He now has cultivated free-style locks, sort of like Caesar, Huey Freeman's buddy in Aaron Magruder's *Boondocks* comic strip.

Roland likes his hair, and lots of other people do too. Strangers often ask him how he does it, or compliment it. They think it's cool. Some kids at school aren't fond of locks or nappiness and crack wise about his hair, but this only makes Roland sigh in bored amusement, because as he says, "Well, du-u-uh! So my hair is nappy! Do I look like I'm embarrassed about nappy hair?"

Roland says, "I feel great about wearing locks. Because I'm the only kid in my whole [elementary] school who wears locks. Um, what's it like? You have to have some skills because you get teased a lot and some kids say stuff like 'your hair is nappy and it looks like worms.' You have to think up good comebacks like 'Your shoes are so old and small that your toes are pokin' through; you look like you're wearing sandals.' I get compliments too though; it's about fifty-fifty. I still wear locks because I just like them. Right now, I just want to say that if you're tenderheaded, do not get your locks twisted because it's going to be painful."

I know that many African American children parrot insults and slights overheard from their parents. They aren't sure why the parents don't approve of or like locked hair but they—at least when young—instinctively want the approval of their parents and so they repeat the attitudes with which they are most familiar. Then, later, when they become more self-confident and see how locked hair has flourished, some of these same children want to know how to grow locks. I had talked the talk, but my son showed me how to walk the walk.

Perhaps Roland will one day decide to cut his locks, but it won't be because he is afraid to wear them. It will be because he has made another hair choice that celebrates his spirit.

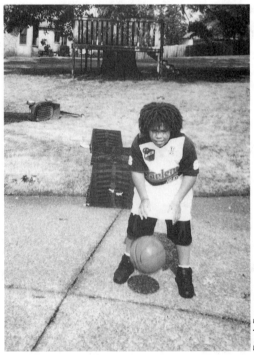

Derek Bonner

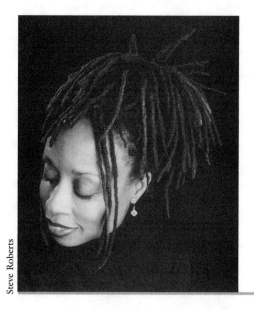

Steve Roberts

# Nine

## Love and Nappiness: Hair Inspiration

I'd spent many years of my life waiting for my hair to catch up to my fantasy of what it should be, and I'd wasted time. I'd structured my lifestyle around my hairstyle. Many women talk about courage, the courage one needs in order to lock one's hair. One of my earliest head trips was the fear of looking like a homeless person about the head, and I felt it was important to make the distinction before my people did. The irony was that no matter how well groomed, clean smelling, charmingly coiled with wayward haphazard little naps escaping it was, my hair was still nappy and therefore ugly. Plenty of women took great comfort in what they viewed as my unattractiveness. Women with hairlines shiny bald from relaxer mishaps, women with hair gelled into hardened towers of waves with baby hair that appeared to have been sketched in with a Sharpie pen, women with bad wigs, women who were passing for Indian as part of the Korean Cherokee tribe, women with transparent hair, brittle snatch backs and wraps hidden under do rags, fingernails digging into scalps that clearly hadn't seen water in a couple of weeks would stand next to me in the hair product aisle and openly eyeball me in amazement, thinking Why are you over here? They meant, You don't need hair care products.

As virulently negative as some of the women were, their menfolk didn't appear to have the same outlook. Many was the time a brother approached me to ask how long I'd been dreading or if was I starting dreadlocks. These men went on to inquire what sort of products I was using and had I done the locks myself. Of course there may have been other motives for the interest—but the point, which was lost on the womenfolk, is that my hair was no deterrent to male interest and in fact was used as a relatively safe conversational opener.

How could I, in all good sense, allow women who didn't have a clue make me feel self-conscious? Well, I suppose you could call it courage, but I simply call it getting my back up. I'd come too long and too far to be swayed by the Losers of the Lost Tribe.

Locks have allowed me to achieve the Impossible Dream: hair that fits my lifestyle, is attractive, and grows like a bat out of Hades. All because I chose to embrace the coil instead of running harder and faster than Sweetback to get away from it.

## THE EYE OF THE BEHOLDER

I've always admired beautifully kept locks and am fascinated with their allure. I craved seeing images of locks worn by fashionable, artistic, professional, creative women. Women with locked hair in various stages of development can now be seen in commercial advertisements for blue-chip corporations, fashion magazines, newspaper stories, comic strips, and greeting cards—thankfully, the list is endless. And so are the possibilities for surrounding yourself with inspiration. When I come across any image of locks that strikes my fancy, I clip it and pin it to the cork bulletin board I call my Lock Wall. I've been doing this for years and now have a collage of inspiration in my office that I can glance at any time I like. Of course, I can glance at my own shoulder-length locks too.

My other inspiration is knowing and meeting women who celebrate their locked hair. Some of these stunning, accomplished women who exemplify the diversity of locks have chosen to share part of their locking experience, while others have chosen simply to share their images, their visual inspiration.

My sister-in-law Capril Bonner-Thomas and her daughter, my niece Maya, were early inspirations for my journey. They shared their early experiences in my book *Plaited Glory: For Colored Girls Who've Considered Braids, Locks, and Twists.* It is a special delight for me that their images are in *Nice Dreads,* and that both mother and daughter continue to celebrate locked hair as a woman in her prime and her daughter, now a young woman.

What I found most poignant is that all the women I've encountered have described their decision to lock their hair as a journey, a liberation, an act of compassion in the interest of their beauty.

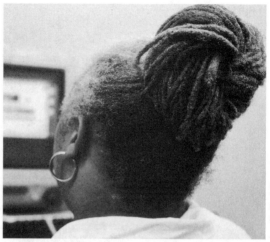

Aurelio José Barrera

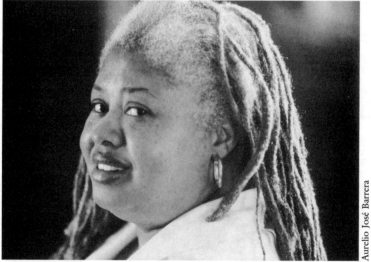

Aurelio José Barrera

## Capril Bonner-Thomas

Quilting artist and designer, book store manager, mother, wife

## Maya Bonner-Thomas

Student, artist, writer

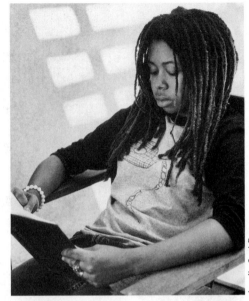

Aurelio José Barrera

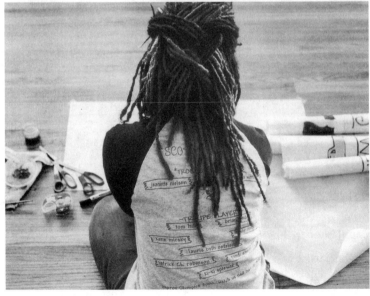

Aurelio José Barrera

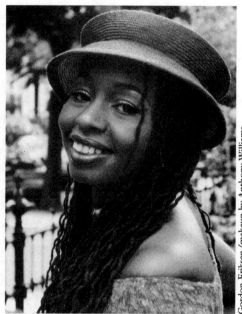

Gordon Eriksen/makeup by Anthony Williams

**Linda Heppard, 52**

**Licensed massage therapist, raw food caterer, herbalist**

**Began locking in 1996**

I began locking my hair seven years ago, being tired of the long sessions of getting micro braids which took sometimes twenty-four hours. I went to a loctician who cared for my hair for about six months; then I began to maintain them myself with the help of what I learned studying herbs and nutrients. I use different natural oils when I twist them, which helps to keep them in place. Many thanks to [loctician] Ruth Borie. Her compassion and concern truly helped me learn how to take care of my hair.

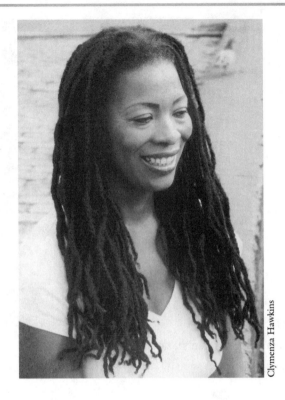

Clymenza Hawkins

**Clymenza Hawkins, 48**
Visual artist, writer, designer, producer, mother
Began locking in 1996

For almost a decade I'd worn my hair in thin braid extensions. When natural locks began becoming popular, my
friends who locked their hair always encouraged me to do
the same because my hair was natural for it. My hair never
took to relaxers very well. My hairline would be straight

but the top was bushy. I knew "locks" were connected to "dreadlocks," and I knew the political history behind it. But a fellow sister understood my hesitation, yet said "Just look at it as a celebration of your natural hair." By the time I wanted to lock my hair, it had already started to lock; I'd let my braid extensions grow out and the new growth had locked and grown over my braids. I went to Locks and Chops (a natural hair salon in Brooklyn) [and asked them] to get rid of the extensions but to save the locks. It's the best thing I've ever done for myself.

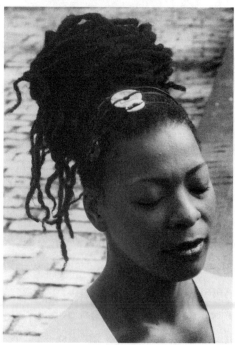

Gordon Eriksen/makeup by Anthony Williams

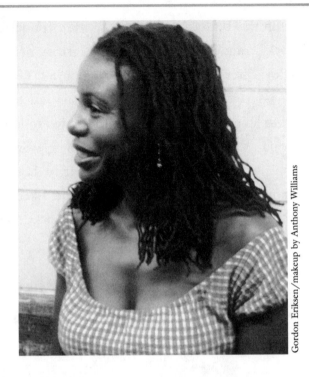

Gordon Eriksen/makeup by Anthony Williams

**Dawne Simon-Ponte, 38**
Attorney, wife, mother
Began locking in 1998

I started locking my hair five and a half years ago. I was pregnant with my son, Diallo, and decided it was time to make the transition. I had been moving toward it for some time. I had thought about locking my hair for at least one to two years before actually taking action. I had gone natural and was wearing a short natural style for about four years before locking my hair. When I decided to lock, I went to a salon and stylist Debra Ottley coiled my hair. I went back about three times before they locked. I was fortunate that my hair locked when it did because I was placed on bed rest for the rest of my pregnancy. Having my hair locked was a blessing because my hair did not suffer the abuse of being in bed for five months.

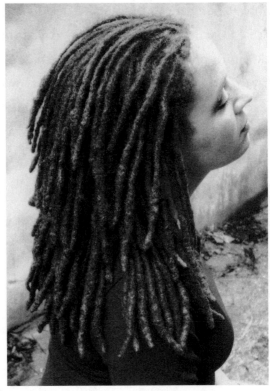

Gordon Eriksen/makeup by Anthony Williams

**Heather Johnston**
Writer, filmmaker, director, wife, mother
Began locking in 2000

I've been wearing my hair natural ever since my daughter
Erica—she's six—was born. Back then, I wore my hair in
braids. Then, when I was pregnant with my daughter
Margo, I took them out and wore a long natural [freedom

'fro]. I didn't like the way I looked in a natural; I guess I was ready because I wasn't afraid to cut my hair really short and start over again. So I went to a salon, Khamit Kinks, and the stylist coiled my hair. I went back six weeks later, and she pulled out a coil and it had already started to bud; they didn't wash out. It was pretty fast.

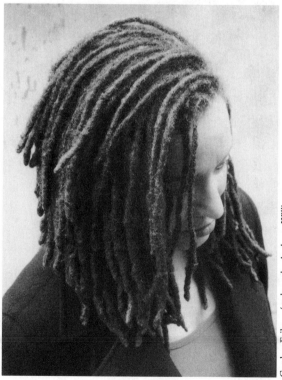

Gordon Eriksen/makeup by Anthony Williams

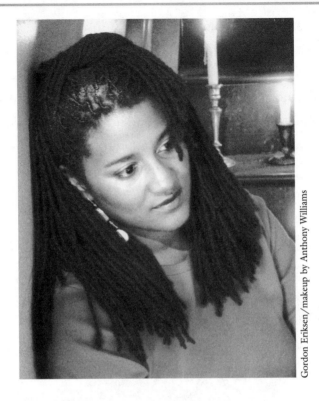

Gordon Eriksen/makeup by Anthony Williams

**Lynn Nottage**
Playwright, wife, mother
Began locking in 1993

I was transitioning out of a job and wanted an entirely new hairstyle to accompany my new lifestyle. I was moving from working as a public relations officer for a large nonprofit into the life of an artist (writer). The locks seemed a way (at the time, few people were locking) to assert my independence.

I went to a hairstylist who did the initial twisting of my hair, which was incredibly short at the time. After that, I've continued the maintenance until now. I've cut my locks three times since then, primarily because the length was causing back pain. Each time I cut my hair, I found that my life took huge leaps forward.

*Author's note: I must add that Lynn is not exaggerating about the length and lush weight of her locks, which when I first met her were well past her waist. I am glad she continues to lock her hair because it is fabulous!*

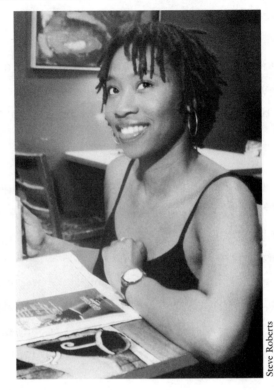

Steve Roberts

**Tonya Meeks**
Paralegal, yoga teacher
Began locking in 2002

My father championed my hair even when it was in the budding stage. He called me his "little rebel daughter." My relatives in Memphis were not as enthusiastic—they were worried about my job—but my boss has complimented my hair.

I take a holistic approach when it comes to taking care of my hair. I eat nutritionally, and I treat my hair the same way. I use natural oils like rosemary and almond and shampoo it with Dr. Bronner's. I shampoo whenever it feels dirty—in summer, that might mean as many as three times a week, and in winter, maybe once a week. I prefer to maintain my locks myself, although I started them with Indigo [a Memphis loctician]. People have asked questions about my hair, can I wash it, etc., but it doesn't bother me. It's just part of the journey.

I've received many more compliments all around since I began locking, except from some black women. They stressed how unattractive I would be to men if I had natural hair, but that has not been the case. I've felt greatly liberated wearing natural hair. I started out wearing a close-cropped 'fro, then twists, and then I began locking. It's never been better. My mother is thinking about locking her hair as well.

Locking my hair has made me feel much more confident and attractive; it's been extremely gratifying emotionally. In the past year, I've observed many fascinating changes in my hair as the locking process has continued. Now that my hair is longer, I feel even more feminine, and I think my hair is more beautiful now than ever.

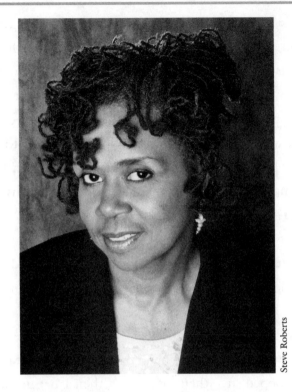

Steve Roberts

**Cassandra Hughes Webster**
Marketing/communications consultant, serves on several boards
that impact the lives of women and children; wife and mother
Began locking in 2001

I've worn my hair long, short, and in braids, every which
way. I began wearing Sisterlocks in 2001 and never looked
back. It's been such freedom. My daughter, McKenzii, has
never had a relaxer, and the hair experience was our weekly

challenge due to her active schedule. So she decided she wanted Sisterlocks too. It was so liberating for her. She says, "I love my hair, it makes me uniquely me."

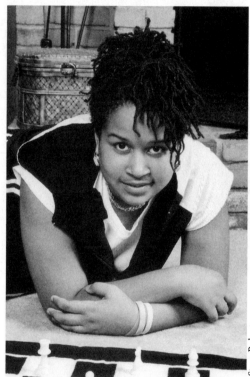

Steve Roberts

**McKenzii Denise Webster**

Thirteen-year-old honors student, attends a science and engineering academy in Memphis, Tennessee; plays guitar, piano, chess, and basketball

I'm continually amazed at the comments from people re-garding my Sisterlocks. It ranges from "Ooh, they're so beautiful! I wish I had the nerve to do that!" to "You obvi-ously don't work for Corporate America." I just chuckle and respond, "I work with corporations all the time."

In my opinion, it's about how you carry yourself. It's your message, it's your business savvy, it's the total package. Sisterlocks have a cultural polish that simply works for me.

## A MEMBER OF THE CLUB

I began growing my locks in 2000. Almost from the beginning, I got encouragement and compliments from people who asked if I were starting locks. The majority of discouragement came from black women who cloaked their derision by asking how long I was going to wear my hair "that way" or how I got my hair "like that."

**Vea Williams**

**Singer, actress, songwriter**

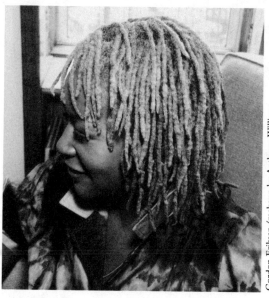

Gordon Eriksen/makeup by Anthony Williams

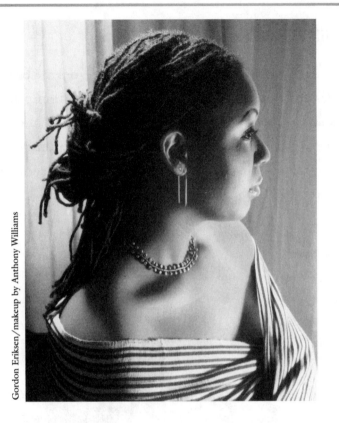

Gordon Eriksen/makeup by Anthony Williams

**Erica Simone Turnipseed**
Novelist, philanthropist

The rap has been that men don't like nappy hair, you won't get a man with your hair like that. Yes, there are men who can't stand hair that is not straight or straightened, who will lust after the fabled good hair until they die. I couldn't compete in the good hair competition, so those guys weren't after me in the first place. That's life, but this is reality: Women who wear locks universally agree they've never gotten more compliments in their lives. I can testify to this, totally.

When my locks were sprouting, I could separate the ne'er-do-wells from the true lovers of coiled hair. As my

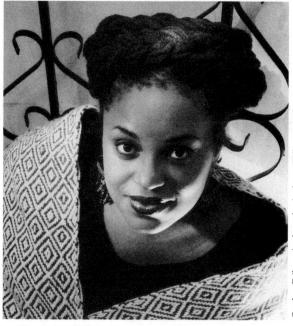

Gordon Eriksen/makeup by Anthony Williams

**Nicole Payen**
Professor, writer, wife, mother

hair became longer, plenty of people jumped on the band-wagon. Instead of focusing on the few negative feelings or comments, think about how your life will change once your locks begin to flourish. I remember the wonder I felt when I noticed that the locks that had formerly framed my forehead in bangs had crept down past my jawline; they would swing toward my fork at mealtimes, so I had to push it out of the way. Once my hair had grown past my shoulders it stayed out of the way for the most part, but the shorter, shoulder-length pieces still swing across my face.

It was then that I realized just how my locks had grown, an experience I had never expected. It is one thing to fling extensions over one's shoulder, but to have the pleasure of feeling one's own hair—delicious!

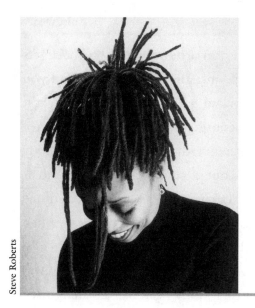

Steve Roberts

# Ten

## Your New Life as a Locked-Hair Diva

Imagine, your hair waist length! Not a false hair extension but your own hair, grown naturally, without a remarkable fast-acting formulation, and you are at your wit's end trying to manage it! Incredible but true!

Who would have thought the day would come when you would actually complain about your *hair*—not your braid extensions, not your weave, not your wig, but your own hair, being . . . in your way . . . a nuisance to sleep on . . . you have to gather it out of the way so you can sit down.

When someone puts an arm around you, your hair gets pulled . . . it dips into your plate when you eat and you have to make sure it is pulled back . . . you must protect it in inclement weather, contrary to your past visions of traipsing through the street with it blowing in the windy cold . . . you sling it back out of your eyes, over your shoulder, just the way you used to when you stood in front of the mirror with a towel over your head pretending you had long hair.

The first time I realized my hair was Officially Long was while driving my car. I turned my head while leaning back in my seat and felt a firm tug because I was leaning back against my hair, which had crept past my shoulderblades.

You have become your fantasy, your dream.

I thought I knew how to handle long hair because I'd worn extensions before. But managing braid extensions and weaves were child's play. I certainly wasn't worried about them breaking off; my concern was figuring out how to make the mass of extensions look credible so people wouldn't roll their eyes and call me "Lady Godiva" behind my back. Learning how to manage long hair is a tiny bit of an adjustment, but once you get into the groove you'll never look back.

## SOME POINTS TO KEEP IN MIND

- Be aware of your hair around car doors and doors in general.
- Take care around candles, lighters, and other sources of fire.
- Bring your hair to the front of your shoulders on each side before putting on your coat.
- When dancing with a partner, have him put his arm under your hair because if he leans on it the pressure can strain your neck and stress your hairline at the temples and nape.
- If your partner sweeps you off your feet and into his arms, bring your hair forward over your shoulders; again, this will prevent accidental tugging and pulling.

Enjoy your locks. Life is too short not to.

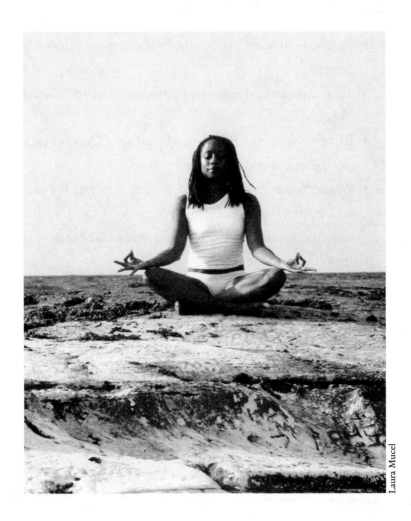

# resources

**nappturality.com**
**naani.com**
There is a marvelous community of coily-haired people and information out in cyberspace. One of the stellar sites is **naani.com,** and **nappturality.com** has an excellent listing of links for coily hair Web sites.

**Intertwined**
An annual locked hair conference based in Brooklyn, New York, founded by expert loctician Nekhena Evans. Well worth attending,

especially if you're out in the boondocks and need inspiration and validation, not to mention being surrounded by beautiful heads of locks of every shape, size, color, age, gender. Products galore, clothing, workshops, entertainment, holistic services. Check it out. New Bein' Enterprises. www.newbein.com. P.O. Box 400106, Brooklyn, NY 11240-0106. Tel. 718-638-5725.

## Sisterlocks.com

"Sisterlocks is not about a hairdo. It's about a way of life!" states Sisterlocks creator, Dr. Joanne Cornwell, in her promotional booklet for Sisterlocks consultants. The Web site has an informative Q&A page for those considering the sisterhood.

## Latching

Another method of starting extra-small locks is called *latching*, and it is *similar* to the Sisterlocks technique. Latching involves using a latch hook (which can be purchased at most craft and sewing supply stores) to interlock hair into a chain link. An excellent resource is an instructional book titled *How to Retighten Your Locs Using the Latchin' Technique,* by Cherie M. King. Crowning Glory Natural Hair e-Publications, Detroit, MI. Tel. 800-304-7025. http://herspecialhair.com.

## PRODUCTS

*I have used these nationally distributed products and like them.*

- **Aveda** Clarifying Shampoo. www.aveda.com.
- **Organic Root Stimulator** (shampoos, conditioners, scalp oils, oil moisturizing lotions). Namaste Laboratories, Blue Island, IL.

## Also by Lonnice Brittenum Bonner

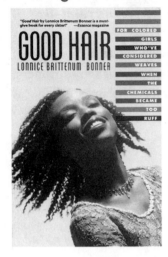

More than a guide to having good hair without relying on harsh treatments and chemicals, *Good Hair* is a funny, folksy, personal, and very wise reflection on the powerful role that hair can play in creating a positive self-image.

0-517-88151-9
$9.95 (Canada: $14.95)

Braids, locks, and twists—from the uptown micro braid to the simple cornrow—have come into their own. *Plaited Glory* gives the lowdown on everything from choosing a braiding salon to differentiating between styles and their costs. More than a "hair do" book, this is a hair primer with a cultural twist.

0-517-88498-4
$12.00 (Canada: $18.00)

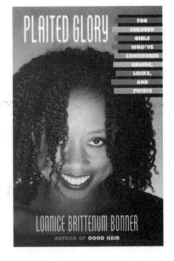